Acup
(heal yourself)

... That any-one can learn for common ailments and effectively utilise Any time, Any place. No tools. No medicine...

Dr. R.P. Gupta

HEALTH 🌳 HARMONY

Printed in India

© With the Author

First Edition : 1995
Reprint Edition : 1996, 1998, 1999, 2001, 2002, 2005

Published by: **HEALTH & HARMONY**
B. Jain Publishers (P) Ltd.
1921, Street No. 10th Chuna Mandi,
Paharganj, New Delhi-110055 (INDIA)
Ph: 2358 0800, 2358 1100, 2358 1300, 2358 3100
Fax: 011-2358 0471; Email: bjain@vsnl.com
Website: www.bjainbooks.com

Printed in India by
J.J. Offset Printers
522, FIE, Patpar Ganj, Delhi - 110 092
Phones: 22169633, 22156128

Book Code : BG 5122
ISBN 81-7021-548-X

A NOTE TO THE READER

The ideas, procedures and suggestions given in this book are not intended to be a substitute for "Acupuncture" or any other conventional therapy. Acupressure is a step towards the body fitness and to develop resistance against body stress, strain and sickness. It should not be understood as a complete cure or in any way, to replace or negate the medical science. Acupressure shall be exercised as a supplement for preventive measures against sickness.

Readers and active participants are advised to consult their physician or an authorized acupuncturist for all health related matters.

This book is intended to help the average person to return to health by natural means. It is designed to show him how to ease his daily ailments and promote well being. This book does not make you a doctor nor does it gives you the know-how or the right to heal people who are seriously ill. Certain points at the end of a few chapters are left blank for further additions.

Comments and suggestions for further improvement will be highly appreciated.

CONTENTS

Introduction	3
Preface	5
1. Applications of Acupressure	11
2. Landmarks	23
3. Critical Points	29
4. Relief Points	35
4.1 Head	39
4.2 Face	45
4.3 Neck	55
4.4 Shoulders and Hands	59
4.5 Chest and Abdomen	75
4.6 Back	89
4.7 Legs	101
5. Acupressure for Maintaining good Health	119
6. Precautions	127
7. Abbreviations	131
8. Index	133
9. Glossary	149
Bibliography	161

INTRODUCTION

In the beginning of my career as Irrigation Engineer my headquarters were in villages and small towns (all along the canals) where medical aid of any kind was hardly available. It created no problem for me or my family as my wife (registered Homoeopath) used to look after this aspect. Besides our family, she had also extended this service voluntarily and freely to the nearby villages. While it helped her to maintain and improve her practice, it developed a very harmonious atmosphere for us among the villagers who consequently looked after our security, welfare, etc. Thus, naturally I developed an interest in Homoeopathy & other simple means of healing such as Naturopathy, Acupressure, etc. As the years passed, it became infact the hobby of not only my wife and myself but that of my family as a whole and we continued the same during our stay in bigger towns/cities also. During the last thirty years, we have gained good knowledge through books and good experience through friendly/free healing practice. After my retirement from Government service, it became almost my whole time utilization through which I had the utmost job-satisfaction and gratification as well.

During my stay in United States, I didn't have a

full time employment. So I was advised by my well-wishers to utilize some of my time in writing a book on Homoeopathy or Acupressure based upon my long practical experiences. It also appealed me and accordingly I decided to give their suggestion a practical shape.

It is in this way, that this book has come into existence. While writing, I have made all efforts to use easy to understand language and to write a concise but complete book helpful in common ailments troubling our people all the days in far off areas where, practically, no proper medical aid is readily available or many of them are not in a position to go in time to the places where this medical aid is available.

As I belong to and have been for major part of my life in such areas/people, I know and understand their needs for a book which may serve them as a timely friend in providing healing aids. Hence this book is purely based on their requirements and years of my actual experience of the Acupressure Therapy, aim of which is to restore person's health, balance and harmony at all levels – physical, mental, emotional and spiritual–by stimulating the body's own self-healing powers in a simple and easy-to-do way.

In writing this book, it has been my good fortune to be in America and surrounded by the people most advanced in life and very good in human character. The quality of these persons has not only touched me but also helped me a lot to shape this book to this extent.

PREFACE

Did you ever notice on a bus, at a party or at a place of work that most people do not have a smile on their faces? Did you also ever notice in yourself or others around you that by the end of a working day, really much energy is not left to do some of those personal or family things you really would like to do?

You might have seen that a lot of people are walking around only partly energized as there seems to be something continuously draining them ! Why so?

Remember when you were little and in pain, your mother or father would ask "where does it hurt"? You would tell them, and they could help you to feel better. Now, over the years, through the wear and tear of everyday life, you find it less easy to locate and heal the pain. Then, if you awake one morning with muscle pain or headache, what would your first thought be? Get an aspirin, a tranquilizer or a doctor? Health care is changing. Today we are witnessing a revision of attitudes towards health care that is taking us back in time to more personalized form of health care and ahead towards new ways of viewing health and healing.

Health care varies from time to time, from culture to culture and from country to country. In good old days, Chinese method of healing included treatment with herbs, diet, massage, exercises, etc., but later these methods of treatment were used in conjunction with Acupuncture or even instead of it. In China itself thousands of men and women, the so called "BARE FOOTED DOCTORS", have been trained to look after, relieve, or cure the complaints and ailments of their own families, their neighbours and fellow workers simply by stimulating certain selected points on the body by hand. Similarly in Japan, Shiatsu is a system of body work that uses gentle manipulations combined with finger and hand pressure on the body's energy meridians. By releasing blocked energy, Shiatsu relieves pain and tension, corrects functioning of the internal organs and treats specific conditions of illness. It follows almost the same principles as Chinese healing method of Acupuncture but Acupuncture uses needles, while Shiatsu and acupressure use hand and finger pressure only. Acupressure has, in fact, been called as "Acupuncture without needles".

Acupressure and Shiatsu are often mentioned together, their philosophies both outline an orient perspective on healing. They differ in that Shiatsu may include certain body manipulations, whereas Acupressure, like Acupuncture rests solely on the stimulation of certain points on energy meridians. The original approach to acupressure by practitioners was based entirely on an instinctive knowledge of where to touch and where to press or stimulate.

Nature has designed your marvelous body to serve you efficiently for many years. To assume the same, it has provided built-in systems for normal continuity of vital functions, self maintenance and self healing, which include anti-bodies, blood clotting, a variety of shock absorbers, equalizers, separate brain flows, reserves of eye sight and other facilities. Most important self healer of systemic problems is natural rest. Proper rest/sleep regenerates broken cells, revitalizes elements of life, corrects inner imbalances, regains depleted strength, mental composure, etc. Among the marvelous processes in your inner self are the steps that change what you breath, drink and eat in your body's fuels. Abuses of this system such as over indulgence bring indigestion and cause headache, nausea, constipation, etc. which work as signals for the problems to happen.

Another fascinating inner wonder is the intricate network of tiny currents known as energy flows. These miniature streams of power are integral parts of your nerve and muscle system and cover every inch of your body to ensure proper operation in all normal functions, internally such as disposition and externally such as appearance. These tiny conductors of bodily power control, notify you when any of the systems are not operating within allowable limits. A headache, for example, warns you of an abnormal condition in your head or some times even in any other part of your body system.

In other words, compare your these energy flows to the circuit breakers in the electrical wiring of your home. When a circuit is over loaded the breakers shut off the current to areas served by connected wiring. In our personal power load system we are warned of any abnormal condition or blockage by our small feelings and sometimes by pain to attend them. Usually the congestion spots become painful rather than just sensitive to your touch and are, thus, located easily to work as relief points.

It is considered that the pain or ailment is due to the blockage of energy flow somewhere in the meridian. By pressing or stimulating a certain relief point, this blockage of energy flow is reduced or removed, thus, alleviating the pain of ailment. If the blockage of energy flow is at a juncture of two or more meridians, then any one of the several relief points on these connecting meridians can be effective to eliminate the energy blockage and consequently healing the pain or ailment. Similarly, a relief point on juncture of several meridians can eliminate several pains/ailments. These meridians pass through many parts of the body and connect all vital organs, that is why a "long distance treatment", or pressing a relief point far from the origin of complaint is effective to alleviate the pain.

These methods alone or combined with some personal observations and adjustments can be worked on our bodies in a natural way while relaxing in our homes, watching T.V., doing some light work such as chit-chat or when we are in journey, and gain the extra "plus" – feeling good or better.

Well, that is what this book is about – trying to use some simple methods to make and feel you healthy enough even at the end of the day.

It is hoped that the following chapters will give all details what can be expected to follow a course of Acupressure treatment. They outline the technique, how to find and decide a particular relief point for the specific condition/ailment in a person, how to locate and work out the same, when and how it can be gainfully utilized, etc.

Acupressure is a technique which anyone can learn and apply to himself and to others easily, but as it is true with any other technique, insufficient practice or half knowledge of the subject may not relieve the problems. The effective results will be obtained when the treatment is given by a trained and experienced practitioner or by a person who has acquired thorough knowledge of the subject and its techniques. After you have gone through the book and studied carefully all the concerned/required details, it is hoped your interest in the subject of Acupressure will be enhanced. It is definite that the benefits, which this simple but effective method can so often have, will be more and more with the length of practical experience and the depth of desire you have to help/serve others.

PRACTICAL APPLICATIONS OF ACUPRESSURE

1.
PRACTICAL APPLICATIONS OF ACUPRESSURE

The person applying the acupressure may be doing so either for himself or herself or for an other person. In all the cases, before taking any action for healing, various details regarding the ailment and patient are required to be known through visual supervision, physical examination, consultation, etc. A few of them are given below for example and guidance.

1. At what age or stage did the ailment first become a problem?
2. Did it begin to behave so gradually or suddenly?
3. Was it due to some other ailment or pain or created itself some other pain or ailment?
4. Since its reception, has it increased or decreased? If yes, when, to what extent and for how much duration, etc.

5. What is the actual location of pain in the body?
6. Is it deep in the body or on the surface only, sharp or dull, drilling or knife like, throbbing or just pressing or what is the exact nature of ailment?
7. What are the other associated symptoms which happened before, during and after the happening of this ailment? These may be such as watery eyes, running or blocked nose, red or blotchy face, vomiting or feeling anything else likewise ?
8. What relieves/reduces the pain or makes it worse? Does the pain increase/decrease due to coughing, sneezing, drinking or eating something or wearing tight or loose clothes etc.? If yes, to what extent?
9. Personal or family or locality factors that affect the ailment or patient.
10. Some other essential data such as serious physical or mental injury such as blow on the head or elsewhere, any surgery undergone, recent changes in diet and their effect on ailment, history of any fainting spell or any such event happened recently or far back in past and its effect on body, mind, ailment, etc.
11. Smoking or use of tobacco, drugs, or anything else likewise?
12. Usual or unusual sensitivity or allergy to anything?

Now having gone through all the above information, physical examination, some special tests such as eye-sight or blood tests and, if required, X-rays, EEG, etc. to help the diagnosis, a careful decision is taken up for further action regarding adoption of acupressure and the way it has to be carried out.

The practitioner as well as the patient have to make sure that no abrupt decision or action is taken for which one has to repent later.

The main steps to be carried out practically to accomplish the acupressure gains are :-

(a) To identify a relief point which is required to be worked for a specific condition, pain or ailment.

(b) To locate exactly the relief point on the body part(s).

(c) To activate the concerned relief point by applying suitable massage or pressure techniques.

Each step has now been explained separately in detail in the proceeding paragraphs.

A. Identification of Relief Points:

The relief points, based mainly on their locations on different body parts such as head, face, neck, shoulders, hands, chest, abdomen, back, legs, etc., have been described in separate chapters, and with a serial number against each relief point, the specific conditions, pains or ailments, for which it can be individually and effectively used, are also given.

Based on the specific condition, pain or ailment of the patient, the reader or practitioner may look into the index and select one, two or more relief points and note down their numbers and against the concerned relief points, he or she will check up the ailment for further confirmation and study the details of location for further action.

B. How to Locate a Relief Point:

Bodies of all people are not equal in size, they may be tall or short, fat or thin; hence the same unit of measurement can not be used on all bodies for locating the relief points. It is seen that bodies and their parts are almost proportional to each other. Hence a new unit of measurement called Acupressure-Inch (AI) is deduced separately for each and every person based on the ratio-proportion of his or her body parts. It may be seen that:

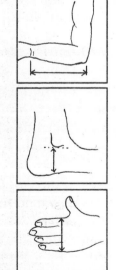

I. The distance from mid-point of eye-brows to the highest point at natural hair line at forehead is equal to 3 AIs.

II. The distance from the farthest wrist fold to the outer corner point of bent elbow is equal to 12 AIs.

III. The distance of highest point on ankle bone on the outer side of feet to the bottom of hell is 3 AIs, and

IV. The width of four fingers measured across the knuckles is 3 AIs.

Keeping any one or all these measurements in view, the actual length of Acupressure-Inch (AI) can easily be estimated for a particular body.

Now based on the given direction and distances in AIs with reference to well-defined body marks, called "Landmarks", explained separately in Chapter 2, exact relief points can be located and marked on the body for further action.

C. How to Activate the Relief Points:

I. Touch the relief point, thus traced/located on the body with the tip of your index finger. Certain portions of skin, particularly in case of children and ladies, are so soft and sensitive that hardly any pressure is required, only touch with small rotations in clock wise/anti-clockwise direction is enough to activate the relief point. Continue the touch for a minute or so.

II. In case simple touching is not considered enough, apply gentle pressure which the patient can bear comfortably. Massage the relief point with your finger in a small clockwise/anti-clockwise circular movement, about two or three cycles per second. The relief points are either single on the central line of the body or double, one point on each side of the central line and at similar position or location on the body. It is preferable to apply pressure bilaterally. Start with one point at a time and attend both the points one after the other. Keep on asking the patient the questions such as:

❏ What are your feeling ?
❏ Are you comfortable ?
❏ Are you feeling better or not ?
❏ etc.

III. If the skin is harder, apply more force, either by

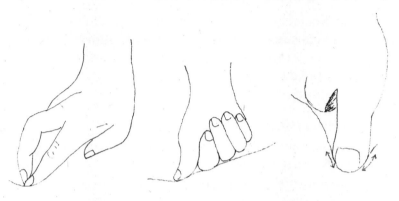

doubling up with your middle finger on top of your index finger or with your thumb alone. The pressure is to be increased gradually to the extent the patient can comfortably afford and keep on asking the questions as indicated in item II hereinbefore. Do not increase the pressure beyond patient's comfort/tolerance limit. Now keep the pressure steady for 30 to 60 seconds for effective results.

IV. In case, point activation as per item III is found in-effective, 'on and off', approach will work better on for 5 to 7 seconds, off for 2 to 3 seconds, and repeating 7 times only, increasing and decreasing the pressure gradually and applying pressure with the ball of thumb.

V. If the skin at the relief point is still harder and activation as per item IV is not considered effective, one of the following steps may be tried/adopted based on the specific situation:-

(a) Apply very gentle pressure with the rounded nail of your finger or thumb, increasing

Practical Applications of Accupressure 19

        thepressure very slowly and only up to the comfortable tolerance of the patient.

   (b) The pressure can be applied with a small rounded tip of an object such as pencil eraser or handle end of artist's brush or end of cover of ball point pen, etc. having an area of a finger tip precisely about 1/8 inch in diameter of wood, plastic or any other non-conductive material. The end should be completely smooth, rounded and seamless. Be more careful to avoid any discomfort, hurt or injury, etc. to the patient. Comfortable and firm pressure is to be continued for 30 to 45 seconds.

   (c) In case (a) and (b) are considered or found ineffective, apply 'on and off' approach very carefully keeping on–off for 5-2 seconds respectively for a period of 60 seconds at a time and avoiding the jerking or punching effects alltogether.

VI. Alternate method of rhythmic on-off technique with increased/decreased pressure as given in Serial IV and V(c) above, is considered to work better. In this, a pressure up to the tolerance limit of patient is applied firmly for 5 seconds, then it is gradually slackened for 2 seconds without releasing it totally and again pushed.

VII. One of the following techniques may also be used for pressing soothing the relief point or the area of pain as considered suitable:-

   (a) Pressing : Press firmly with the bulb of the thumb, palm or elbow. If needed, make forward/backward motions in case of intensive

Practical Applications of Accupressure

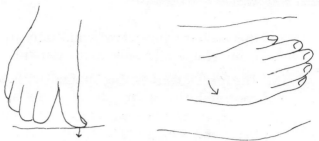

pain in muscles and joints, pressure with elbow is stronger and penetrates more deeply.

(b) Soothing : Use the bulb of the thumb, the fingers or the palm of the hand to massage with light and rapid motion. For more tender and painful areas, this touch can still be lighter and smoother by using a feather. The effect of this

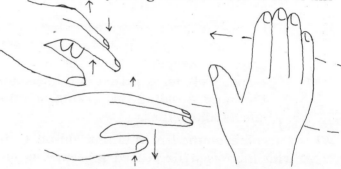

special 'butterfly touch' is electrifying. The body and mind are relaxed and blood starts flowing freely thus relieving the pain.

(c) Pushing : Apply some oil for lubrication and

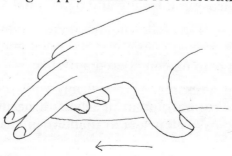

use bulb of the thumb to stimulate or disperse the meridians on the back and the extremities. Pushing is usually applied in series of 100 or more strokes at one time/session.

(d) Picking : Use thumb and index finger to

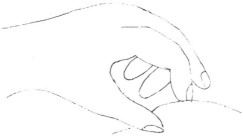

pick-up the skin along with the muscles on the areas such as neck, face, back, etc.

(e) Rubbing : Use the thumbs, fingers and palms of both hands simultaneously to rub the

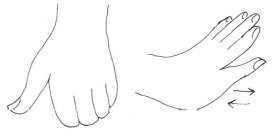

arms and legs, particularly for arthritis, and it will be found very effective.

VIII It may be noted with care that if one of the above techniques is found ineffective, the other technique should not be applied just after on the same relief point. It can be applied only after 8 hours at least.

IX. The degree of pressure may be varied based upon the physique and condition of the subject/patient. Generally light pressure is applied:-

(a) When the subject is child or a women having tender skin.

(b) He or she is getting acupressure for the first time.

(c) When he or she is weak in health or over-tired.

(d) When his/her muscles are weak or loose.

(e) When there is swelling, acute pain or some other complication such as anaemia, heart trouble or high blood pressure, etc.

X. It may also be noted that stimulation, pressing or massage of a relief point should not be continued more than one minute in one session and not more than three sessions per day. If it is done, it may be harmful instead of being useful.

LANDMARKS

2.

LANDMARKS

Certain points are well marked and permanently established on the ground for the purpose of locating other temporary points as and when required. These permanent points are called landmarks. Their records in terms of direction and distance with respect to the specific permanent features is maintained permanently for future references.

Similarly, a point can also be located more easily and correctly if its directions and distances are given with respect to a well known, prominent and easy to find anatomical mark on the body. Here also it is called 'Landmark' for this purpose. A list of such landmarks with their most commonly known names is given as under:

1. Natural hair line on the forehead.
2. An assumed line passing over the head and joining the highest points of two ears.
3. Natural hair line at the back of head and neck.
4. An assumed line passing through the mid points of head and neck, shoulders, back, tail bone, etc.

5. Similarly, an assumed line passing through the mid points of forehead, eye brows, chin, adam's apple on the throat, notch at the base of the throat, chest, naval and genitals.
6. Eyebrows and their both ends.
7. Eyes and their both corners.
8. Nose, its tip, base on both sides, nostrils, etc.
9. Top, bottom and sides of the ears.
10. Two corners of mouth where two lips meet.
11. Centers of both lips.
12. Chin, its center, central and lowest point or line.
13. Adam's apple on and in front of throat.
14. Notch (central depression) at the base of throat.
15. Collar bones and their ends.
16. Spine knob at the neck – the first knob or vertebra more easily visible when head is tilted forward and chin is touching the chest.
17. Arm-pits.
18. Tops of shoulders directly above arm pits.
19. Nipples of breasts and line joining them.
20. Inner and outer elbow folds.
21. Inner and outer wrist folds.
22. Knuckles and joints of thumb and fingers.
23. Navel.
24. Thigh-stomach fold (front side)
25. Buttock fold at the back side.
26. Crease or fold line at the back of knee
27. Knee cap, its top, center and bottom.

Landmarks

28. Inner and outer ankle bone protruding points.
29. Heels, their back, sides and soles.
30. Knuckles, joints and ends of toes.

The details of other body parts. their functions, ailments and their causes are not considered necessary to be included in this book. If needed, readers and practitioners may refer other texts on the subject.

CRITICAL AND IMPORTANT POINTS IN ACUPRESSURE

3.

CRITICAL AND IMPORTANT POINTS IN ACUPRESSURE

1. Acupressure is so effective that often the patient looks amazed how soon the pain has disappeared. It can even rescue people from life long drug-taking habits.
2. Acupressure is medically sound, effective, inexpensive, practical, safe and without any side effects.
3. Before you begin, assure the patient about the effectiveness and success of acupressure in relieving pains without any problem.
4. No tool or special arrangement is required at all.
5. The treatment place must be clean, quiet, and warm, i.e. neither hot nor cold. It should be well ventilated also.

6. One of the best places to give acupressure on back, chest, abdomen, stomach, etc. is a carpeted floor as the firmness of the floor makes it easier for both the patient and the practitioner.
7. While working on back, let the patient lie flat on his stomach with his face turned sideways, never place a pillow under his head as this may produce muscle spasm when pressure is applied to neck and shoulders. His arms should be at his sides and he should not cradle his head in his arms as this position will prevent him from relaxing fully. His rib-cage must rest flat and even on the floor.
8. When working on patient's chest, abdomen, and stomach, he must lie on his back, with arms on sides and pillow under his head. In all positions, patient's mouth should be slightly open and eyes closed for more relaxation.
9. The patient can sit comfortably either on floor, stool or chair when points on his body parts other than back, chest and abdomen are being worked.
10. The patient must be comfortable and totally relaxed because rigid body works as a barrier and prevents any healing from taking place.
11. Use acupressure when patient is relaxing, in a soothing and happy mood, enjoying music on radio or T.V. He MUST NOT be worried or in tension at all.
12. Apply pressure when the patient is exhaling because while inhaling, his body becomes tighter and harder to accept acupressure effectively.
13. Practitioner's thumb and fingers (of hands) and body of the patient should be clean and at same temperature. The practitioner should keep his

nails trimmed to prevent injuring the subject or making him or her nervous and tense.

14. Do not press the point timidly. Work with confidence as this normally leads to excellent results.

15. It may be possible that relatively lighter pressure is enough for one patient while the other may need a little more pressure to make the technique effective.

16. While pressing, consider if you are applying too little or too much pressure as pressing harder may cause some pain. It may also be noted that by no means less force is less effective.

17. An ordinary blunt, round, non-conductor object or finger/thumb nail may be pushed hard enough to effect the underlying nerve but NOT to injure the skin. Avoid working on skin surface where there is contusion, scar or infection.

18. The two points of a pair can be pressed alternately or simultaneously but never neglect one half of the pair even if the pain or problem is only on one side of the body.

19. It is advisable to use watch or clock for measuring the on and off gaps and should not be done merely by guess. It may be continued for a minute or so and repeated only twice (or maximum thrice) a day.

20. All the time be careful about the patient and keep asking him now and then if he/she is comfortable, happy and feeling better or not.

21. Stop treatment if no relief is observed and the symptoms are being aggravated.

RELIEF POINTS FOR HEALING AILMENTS

4.

RELIEF POINTS FOR HEALING AILMENTS

Relief points (RP) are the the keys of acupressure and it is really a challenge for a practitioner to know/learn sufficiently enough how to locate, sense and operate them conveniently and effectively. Though we have tried to give enough description to explain the nature and locations of the relief points in the previous chapter, still, there is something more critically associated with the sensitivity of the relief points which should be clearly understood by every practitioner. A brief description explaining about sensitiveness and how a relief point is associated with the body energy system is presented in the paragraphs given here-in-after.

Relief point is usually a highly sensitive area which often seems to be the size and shape of a fingertip. The hyper-sensitivity of a Relief Point is a signal to the practitioner that energy has stagnated in that part of the body while the rest of the meridian and its associated organs have been cut off that energy supply. This may lead to pain, but not always, extreme stiffness or a highly ticklish feeling at RP may indicate a problem. When ever a light touch produces tremendous pain or hyper-sensitivity at a RP, you can be sure there is trouble somewhere in the body. There are about 1,000 Relief Points along all the meridian lines but only about 300 are most effective. You may ask – why a particular RP on a meridian line is more effective to treat than any other on the same meridian? The answer is that energy has a greater tendency to stagnate in some RPs than in others, although all the RPs on a single meridian are connected to the same area of the body. Therefore, only important RPs which either have quick and relatively high effective response or are related to the common ailments, are described in the proceeding chapters.

For the facility in locating and efficient use, all important RPs have been individually described in detail in chapters based on their anatomical locations. Parts and sub-parts of the body have also been shown in different figures depicting the location of RPs as described with respect to land marks or otherwise. Besides the pressing techniques, ailments for which the specific RP is to be activated, certain clues – more useful to the layman in finding the RPs than the technical anatomical terms, are also given.

RELIEF POINTS ON HEAD

Relief Points on Head

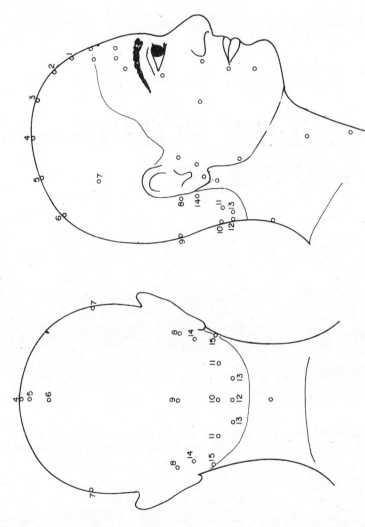

FIG. 1

4.1

RELIEF POINTS ON HEAD

(Refer Fig. 1.)

Relief Point # 1

    Use : For headache, pus or abscess in pleural cavity or gall bladder, nose problems such as sinus, obstruction, bleeding, etc., and hay fever.

    Loc : One point only, on the mid-line of the head. 1 AI behind the front hair-line.

Relief Point # 2

    Use : For headache, dizziness, nose bleeds and colds, problems of stomach, lungs and brain. it helps in absorption of oxygen from blood into the brain.

    Loc : One point only, on the mid-line of the head. 2 AIs behind the front hair-line.

Relief Point # 3

    Use : For headache with a feeling that head will

explode, low blood pressure.

Loc : One point only, on the mid-line of the head, 3.5 AIs behind the front hair line.

Relief Point # 4

Use : For migraine, headache, nose bleed, body shape-up and tinnitus.

Loc : One point only, on the mid-line of the head, 5 AIs behind the front hair-line.

Relief Point # 5

Use : For headache, heatstroke, haemorrhoids, despair and depression, memory deterioration, problems of stomach, heart, abdominal cramps, gas, indigestion, and tingling sensation through body from head to feet.

Loc : One point only, on skull along the line joining the upper edges of the two ears and 6.5 AIs behind the front hair.

Relief Point # 6

Use : For headache, problems of pituitary and pineal glands, brain, colon, enlarged legs, bloat (inflammation) and excess fluid.

Loc : One point only, on the mid-line of head, 8 AIs behind the front hair-line.

Relief Point # 7

Use : For migraine, headache, neck pain, and addiction (all drugs).

Loc : Two points, each on the side of the skull exactly on the line joining highest point of ears and 3 AIs from each ear.

Relief Point # 8

Use : For earache, appetite, brain, toxicity and congestion in the veins, loss of hearing, pain, infection and small boil in ear, motion sickness and insomnia.

Loc : Two points, each just behind the ear. Pull the ear a little forward and find the point in the slight depression near the mastoid bone.

Relief Point # 9

Use : For gas indigestion, brain stroke and pancreas.

Loc : One point only, on the mid-line of head, back of skull and on the line joining the centers of the ears.

Relief point # 10

Use : For mental tension and anxiety, hay fever, low blood pressure, migraine, headaches, common cold, and strokes.

Loc : One point only, in the mid-line of head back and 1 AI above the natural hair-line at back of head.

Relief Point # 11

Use : For common cold, headaches, migraine, fatigue, dizziness, swollen eyes and stiff neck, vomiting, conjunctivitis, teeth and head hurts, deafness tinnitus, face/body shape-up, nose bleeding.

Loc : Two points in depression immediately below the rear head bones, 2 AIs either side of (RP) # 10 and almost at the same level.

Relief Point # 12
- **Use :** For common cold, headache, migraine, nose bleed.
- **Loc :** One point only, on the mid-line of back of head and 0.5 AI above the natural hair-line.

Relief Point # 13
- **Use :** For common cold, nose bleed, nasal obstruction, headaches, migraine, allergies, haemorrhage, and bed wetting.
- **Loc :** Two points, 1.5 AI either side of RP # 12 and almost at the same level, i.e. 0.5 AI above the natural back hair-line.

Relief Point # 14
- **Use :** For inflammation of part or all of the mastoid process and disorders of the intestines, colon and ears.
- **Loc :** Two points, each on a small, raised bone behind the lower portion of ear.

Relief Point # 15
- **Use :** For part or total loss of memory which may be due to shock, psychological disturbance, brain injury or illness, head cold, headache, fatigue of neck, pain in sides of the head, dizziness, deafness, ringing in the ears.
- **Loc :** Two points, each on the slender and pointed/raised bone just below the ear.

RELIEF POINTS ON FACE

Relief Points on Face

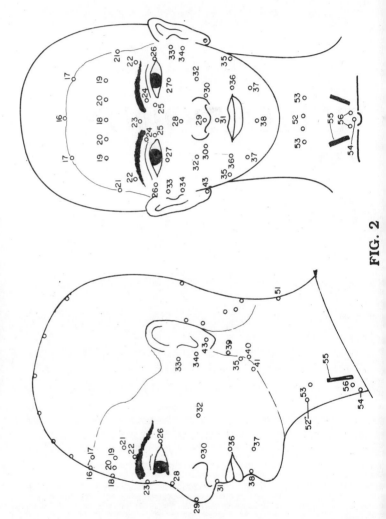

FIG. 2

4.2

RELIEF POINTS ON FACE

(Refer Fig. 2)

Relief Point # 16

Use : For allergies, hay fever, winter ailments, cold/flu, sinus or spasmodic catarrh with sneezing bouts, virus/chronic infection, running or blocked nose, soreness and irritation of eyes.

Loc : One point only, in the middle of forehead hair-line centrally above the bridge of nose near a small bump in a small hollow just beyond the hair-line.

Relief Point # 17

Use : For simple headaches. It energizes face, scalp, forehead and soothes abdomen, gall bladder and liver.

Loc : Two points, on the forehead hair-line just above the eyes pupils when looking straight forward.

Relief Point # 18

Use : For Pituitary gland which affects the chemistry of body.

Loc : One point only, just under Relief Point # 16 and in the very center of the forehead.

Relief Point # 19

Use : Gives energy to face and neck, skin and muscle-tissues which avoid wrinkles, migraine, headache, insomnia, etc.

Loc : Two points just below Relief points # 17, mid-way between hair-line and top of the eyebrow, just above eye pupils when looking straight forward.

Relief Point # 20

Use : For blurred vision, mental conditions.

Loc : Two points, each on the same level and just half-way between Relief Points # 18 and # 19.

Relief Point # 21

Use : For headache, red and swollen eyes, dizziness, tonic for facial muscles, double vision.

Loc : Two points on natural hair-line of forehead 1/2 AI beyond the outer end of the eyebrow and 1 - 1/2 AIs above it and where the hair-line just joins the upper part of the sideburns.

Relief Point # 22

Use : For reduction of development of creases (crow's feet) near eyebrows, tension of shoulders, neck and eyes, headache and breathing problems, visual disturbance, conjunctivitis, eye beautification, glaucoma.

Loc : Two points, at the far end of each eyebrow.

Relief Point # 23

Use : For dizziness, mental tension and anxiety, nasal obstruction, sinus and headache, hypertension.

Loc : One point only, between eyebrows (inside ends).

Relief Point # 24

Use : Eye strain, stomach, hypertension, red and swollen eyes, sinus, sneezing, nasal obstruction, headache and stimulate energy around eyes, face and eye beautification, visual disturbance, glaucoma, blepharites, goiter.

Loc : Two points, at the eyebrows, near nose and inside eye sockets. Treat very gently with thumb-ball (eyes closed).

relief Point # 25

Use : Aching eyes due to a blow, dust and infection such as conjunctivitis, iritis or glaucoma, tension, poor or tired vision and red swollen eyes.

Loc : Two points, each between inner corner of eye and nose base. Treat gently and firmly. Eyes closed.

Relief Point # 26

Use : For irritated and dry eyes, nasal obstruction, running nose, facial tension, headache, wrinkles known as Crow's Feet.

Loc : Two points each 1/2 AI on outer side of the

outer corner of eyes. Treat gently when eyes are closed.

Relief Point # 27
Use : For facial pain, paralysis and tension, tired vision, eye strain, energizes local muscles and tissues, improves sagging skin known as bags below the eyes, sneezing and sinus problems.

Loc : Two points, each below the eyes on the ridge of their sockets, directly below the pupils at the slight depression on the top of the cheek-bone.

Relief Point # 28
Use : It treats pneumonia at its origin and ulcer of duodenum (first 12 inches of small intestine). Press twice daily until improved.

Loc : One point only on top and center of the nose where the bone ends and cartilage begins.

Relief Point # 29
Use : For drugs addiction and for alleviating the effect of over-drinking, electric shock, nose bleed, sneezing.

Loc : One point only on the tip of the nose. Beware, stimulation may cause vomiting.

Relief Point # 30
Use : For nasal obstruction, common cold, allergies, facial tension/paralysis, nose bleed, sinus, running nose, etc., pain on sides of head, pain in stomach, face rejuvenation, conjunctivitis, eye beautification.

Loc : Two points, each on the nose-cheek fold, 1/2

Relief Points on Face

Al up from the bottom of nose on the cheeks.

Relief Point # 31

Use : For loss of consciousness and epilepsy, electric shock, heat/sun-stroke, sinus, sneezing and paralysis (stimulating pituitary gland). Emergency point for fainting, dizziness, nausea, epilepsy, syncope and nose bleeding.

Loc : One point only on the center of upper lip and 1/3 the distance down from the base of the nose to the edge of upper lip.

Relief Point # 32

Use : For toothache, facial pain and tension, sinus, tonic for facial muscles, pain in cheeks, ear wax.

Loc : Two points, each on the face in level with the nostrils in the bony grove under the cheek and directly below the pupils when looking straight forward.

Relief point # 33

Use : For ringing in the ears, disorders of kidney and colon, migraine and tootchache upper jaw.

Loc : Two points. 1/2 Al from front of ear and in the small depression which appears just in front of ear (middle point) when mouth is opened.

Relief Point # 34

Use : Improves blood circulation in heart, body muscles, eyes and works in heart attack: ringing in the ears, sleep disturbance, face-paralysis, dizziness, deafness, earache and toothache.

Loc : Two points, against the hinge of each jaw bone, just below Relief Point # 33 and near the front of the ear.

Relief Point # 35

Use : For tonsillitis, facial pain, toothache of lower jaw, mumps, premature wrinkles, reproductive organs, tension in jaw, enhances energy in entire face, jaw-lock.

Loc : Two points on the big muscle of the lower jaw bone. On tightening the jaws, an identation is felt at the corner of the jaw and slightly inside from the jawbone end of edge.

Relief point # 36

Use : For stomachache, facial tension, wrinkles around mouth, general tension, toothache.

Loc : Two points near the outer corners of mouth, 1/2 AI away from the point where the lips meet.

Relief Point # 37

Use : For toning up the muscles of chin and around the mouth corners, head colds.

Loc : Two points, each midway between chin and lower lip and about 1/4 AI from outer ends/corners of the mouth.

Relief Point # 38

Use : For wrinkles on the chin and tension in lower jaw, channels energy upto mouth and face beyond.

Loc : One point only, at the center of chin and midway lower lip and chin.

Relief Point # 39

Use : For intoxication and glaucoma, cataract, partial or complete loss of vision and fluids in eyes.

Loc : Two points, each on the back of lower jaw bone below each ear.

Relief Point # 40

Use : For problems of intestines.

Loc : Two points, each on the curve of the lower jaw bone below the ear lobe.

Relief Point # 41

Use : For toothache.

Loc : Two points, one under each side and in a notch towards back of underside of the lower jaw bone.

Relief Point # 42

Use : For drowsiness.

Loc : One point only, at the tip of the tongue. Pinch the tip of the tongue with nails of thumb and middle finger or bite gently with front teeth.

Relief Point # 43

Use : For children's convulsions.

Loc : In the center of ear lobe.

RELIEF POINTS ON NECK

Relief Points on Neck

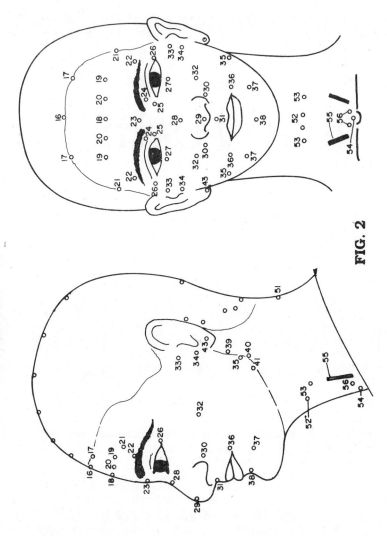

FIG. 2

4.3

RELIEF POINTS ON NECK

(Refer Fig. 2.)

Relief Point # 51

    Use : For problems in the thoracic duct, lymph, chyle and in anaemia.

    Loc : One point only, at the center of the back of the neck about 1-1/2 AIs below the back natural hair line.

Relief Point # 52

    Use : For knee pain, high blood pressure, sore throat, frigidity and thyroid. Generates energy for the whole body, local muscles, tissues on mid-neck throat and face. Restores lost voice.

    Loc : Two points on the throat at the level or slightly above the Adam's Apple and about 1 AI on either side. Massage these points firmly with up and down motion and not hard enough to choke breathing.

Relief Point # 53
  Use : For tinnitus (a defect in auditory nerve)
  Loc : Two points, right at the level of Adam's Apple and 2 AIs on either side of the vertical center line in front of neck/throat. Massage gently with up and down motion.

Relief Point # 54
  Use : For asthma, whiplash, common cold with cough, hoarseness and panting. It gives energy to neck and head.
  Loc : One point only, in the notch of the bone at the base of throat. Be careful not to push into wind pipe. Use index finger to press inward, and massage around softly.

Relief Point # 55
  Use : For thyroid, heart palpitation, weight and body temperature control.
  Loc: Two vertical stretches or strips on each side of front of the neck approximately 1-1/2 AIs at the base and 2 AIs at the top away from central line. Each strip about 1/4 AI in width and 2 AIs in length. Massage with gentle up and down motions.

Relief Point # 56
  Use : Left point works on the left side of the body and heart while right point on the right side of the body and arms.
  Loc : Two points at the front base of the neck and about 1 AI on either side of the vertical center line and about 1 AI above the collar bones.

RELIEF POINTS ON SHOULDERS AND HANDS

Relief Points on Shoulders & Hands

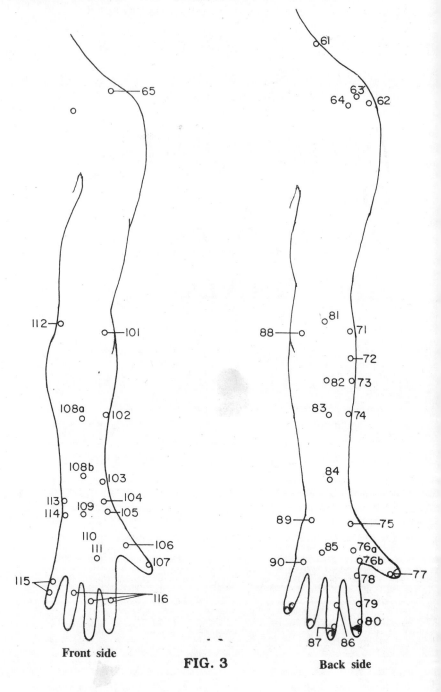

FIG. 3

4.4.1

RELIEF POINTS ON SHOULDERS

(Refer Fig. 3)

Relief Point # 61

Use : For shoulder pain, headache, migraine, fatigue, eye problem, lack of milk in nursing mothers and tension in shoulders and arms; also for cold, asthma, stiff neck, body warmth and energy.

Loc : Two points, each at the shoulder in the hollow formed near the base of neck when the arm is raised. It is vertically directly above the nipple of breast.

Relief Point # 62

Use : For shoulder joint pains, frozen shoulder, bursitis, rheumatoid arthritis.

Loc : Two points, on the top of shoulder in a line vertically above the arm shoulder joint and in a small hollow where the collar bone meets the arm.

Relief Point # 63

Use : For shoulder joint pain, arthritis, elbow pain, hand pain, shock, wounds and cuts.

Loc : Two points, when arm is held horizontally (90 degree to the body), two indentations are formed on shoulder, one on outer side is Relief Point # 62 and the other on the backside is this Relief Point # 63.

Relief Point # 64

Use : For haemorrhage, electric or any other shock and its after effects on heart, concussion, bruises or crushed tissues anywhere on the body, tennis elbow, and exhaustion, apoplexy, all head injuries – how so ever old, and physical fatigue.

Loc : Two points, on the extreme edge of shoulder about 2 AI behind the highest point, in the hollow formed when hand is raised. It is lower and back side of Relief Point # 63. Treat both points left and right simultaneously.

Relief Point # 65

Use : For pains of arms, neck and shoulders, breathing problems and circulation from liver to heart.

Loc : Two points, each just below the outer end of collar bones on shoulders where they meet the shoulder prominence on front side.

4.4.II

RELIEF POINTS ON HANDS

(Refer Fig. 3)

Note : One point is at similar location on each hand and has the same use. Both hand-points are to be treated simultaneously or alternately.

A. Back Side of Hands :

Relief Point # 71

    Use : For any arm problem, diarrhoea, headache, fevers, bursitis, shoulder pain, tennis elbow, rheumatoid arthritis and hypertension.

    Loc : At the depression, a little above the elbow fold (when the elbow is straight) and at the thumb side edge.

Relief Point # 72

    Use : For sore legs, pain and fatigue in the arms, general well being.

    Loc : In depression below the elbow fold at the thumb side edge and 1-1/2 AIs below RP # 71.

Relief Point # 73

Use : For bursitis, indigestion, impotency and premature ejaculation. It works as a tonic for body.

Loc : About 1-1/2 AIs below RP # 72 at the thumb side edge.

Relief Point # 74

Use : For aerophagia (air swallowing), heart-burn, digestion troubles, stomach ulcer, gall-stones, and pain in the chest similar to angina.

Loc : Outside of the upper edge of the fore arm and 4-1/2 AIs from elbow joint towards wrist.

Relief Point # 75

Use : For migraine, headache (very prominent).

Loc : On outer wrist fold, top of hand where hollow is felt at the base of thumb when thumb is stretched.

Relief Point # 76 # A

Use : For diarrhoea, rashes, facial tension, toothache, earache, nose bleed and blocked, red and swollen eyes, common cold, sore throat, elbow pain, migraine, general/whole body arthritis, rheumatoid, sinus, tonsillitis, tinnitus, whiplash, frigidity. Tonic for general health, ankle pain and all headaches, hiccough, head-cold, hay fever, premature ejaculation, conjunctivitis, gingivitis, eye beautification, deafness, ear wax, fatigue of hand, blepharitis, visual disturbance, glaucoma, paralysis of hand and face, insomnia, anxiety, bodyshape-up.

Relief Point # 76-B

Use : For loss or reduction of voice, all ailments of throat.

Loc : At the edge of web between thumb and index finger and about 1½ AI below RP # 76-A.

Relief Point # 77

Use : For sore throat; meningitis at the beginning, rheumatic fever, kidney disease, etc.

Loc : On the side of thumb facing the index finger and just at the base of nail.

Relief Point # 78

Use : For exhaustion, gout.

Loc : Immediately in front of the knuckle and on the thumb side edge of the index finger.

Relief Point # 79

Use : For shoulder pain, diarrhoea, constipation, arm pain.

Loc : On the second or the middle joint and side of index finger towards the thumb.

Relief Point # 80

Use : For bursitis, toothache.

Loc : On the index finger at the intersection of a line drawn along the thumb side edge of nail and a horizontal line across the base of nail.

Relief Point # 81

Use : For pains of head, neck and arms stomachache and acid indigestion.

Loc : Plural contacts on outside aspect of each upper bone, outer side of arm about 4 AIs in length from elbow towards shoulder.

Relief Point # 82

Use : For release of mucous in the body and helps in the circulation of forearm and hand.

Loc : At the point where the two bones begin to spread apart, outer side of arm just 3 AIs down the elbow outer fold.

Relief Point # 83

Use : For chest pains (in heart, lungs, muscles, nerves or ribs), it may be heart attack, angina or pulmonary, or clot in the lungs; for general well being of old people.

Loc : On the middle of back of forearm and almost half way between elbow and wrist.

Relief Point # 84

Use : For colds, aching wrist or hand, constipation.

Loc : About 2-1/2 AIs above wrist fold on the back of forearm and in the middle of width where the two bones meet.

Relief Point # 85

Use : For back and breast pains.

Loc : On the back of hand in between ring and little

fingers and about 4 AIs above the nail of little fingers.

Relief Point # 86

Use : For hic-cough.

Loc : On the middle joint of middle finger and at the edge near index finger.

Relief Point # 87

Use : For mental tension and anxiety, toothache.

Loc : At the nail of middle finger, at the intersection of a line drawn along the index-finger-side edge of the nail and a horizontal line drawn across the base of the base nail.

Relief Point # 88

Use : For sugar control, common cold with fever, elbow pains.

Loc : On the projecting outer corner of the bent elbow.

Relief Point # 89

Use : For pains of wrist and hand.

Loc : On the little finger side, a little beyond the wrist on the second wrist-fold that forms when it is bent outward.

Relief Point # 90

Use : For headache, numbness or paralysis of fingers, hand pain, whiplash.

Loc : On the fold that appears, when the hand is

making a fist, just above the knuckle of little finger, pinch it with nails of thumb and middle finger.

Relief Point # 91

Use : For fainting or loss of consciousness and toothache.

Loc : On the little finger at the intersection of line along the base of nail with vertical line along the ring finger side of nail.

Relief Point # 92

Use : For painful, deformed fingers when one or more fingers are knocked, banged, strained, cut and become unaffected or deformed.

Loc : On the back of the effected finger at its first joint. If all the fingers are effected, stimulate ring finger, thumb, middle finger, index finger and little finger respectively.

Relief Points on Hands (Contd.)

B. Front Side of Hands : (Refer Figure # 3)

Relief Point # 101

    Use : For cough, elbow pain, labored breathing, fever with lung problems, body stiffness, bursitis, tennis elbow, asthma, hic-cough.

    Loc : On inner (body side) of elbow fold 1/2 AI from upper or thumb side edge of arm (right on the crease).

Relief Point # 102

    Use : For cough, shoulder pain, tonsillitis.

    Loc : On the inside surface of forearm, 5 AIs down the inner elbow fold and 1/2 AI from the upper or thumbside edge.

Relief Point # 103

    Use : For common cold, headaches, facial pain, cough, asthma, vertigo, nerve-paralysis, hic-cough, chest pain, paralysis of hands.

    Loc : 2 AI above the inner wrist fold, 1/2 AI from

upper or thumb side edge and near the pulse point. (thumb side).

Relief Point # 104

Use : Painful breathing, cough, pharyngitis (inflammation of Pharynx) relieving unconsciousness, headache, bronchitis.

Loc : 3/4 AI above the inner wrist fold, 1/2 AI from upper edge.

Relief point # 105

Use : For suffocation, uterus and prostate.

Loc : Right on the inner wrist fold 1/2 AI from thumb side edge.

Relief Point # 106

Use : For cough, tonsillitis, hysteria, thyroid.

Loc : 1 AI above from the edge of web between thumb and index finger, on the crease of thumb with the palm near the thumb knuckle

Relief Point # 107

Use : For cough, gingivitis (inflammation of gums), sore throat, nose bleed, sun stroke, painful breathing, pharyngitis, hand spasm, tired arms.

Loc : On the outer side of the thumb, 0.1 AI outer from base of nail.

Relief Point # 108-A

Use : Prolongs youngage and recedes old age.

Relief Points on Hands (Contd.) 71

Loc : One point only, on the center of inner face (side) of right arm, half-way between elbow and wrist folds.

Relief Point # 108-B

Use : For arthritis (general, whole body), shock, nausea, vomiting, insomnia, palpitation: motion-sickness.

Loc : At the center (middle) of two edges, 2.5 AIs up from inner wrist fold on the inner surface of the forearm.

Relief Point # 109

Use : For electric shock, concussion (shock or injury due to violent blow), sunburn or other burns, wrist ailments.

Loc : On the center of inner wrist fold (between Relief Points # 105 and 114).

Relief Point # 110

Use : For suffocating sensation, shivering and perspiration alternately, excitement and despair, fatigue, all signs of depression and sciatica.

Loc : Whole length of inner wrist fold to be rubbed with the thumb of other hand.

Relief Point # 111

Use : For writer's cramp, nose bleed and other problems like exhaustion, frigidity, infertility, excessive sweating, poly-hydrosis, fatigue of hand and solar plexus.

Loc : On the palm where the tip of the completely flexed middle finger touches the middle crease of palm.

Relief Point # 112

Use : For bronchitis, difficult breathing, bursitis, cough, exhaustion, haemorrhage, snake bite, palpitation, elbow pain, paralysis of hand.

Loc : About 1/2 AI above the lower edge (body side) of inner elbow fold.

Relief Point # 113

Use : For shock, migraine headache, mental tension and anxiety, insomnia, toothache, irritability, constipation, obesity.

Loc : 1/4 AI from the lower edge (little finger side) and 1 AI above the inner wrist fold.

Relief Point # 114

Use : For electric shock, fainting, palpitation, irregular heart beat, insomnia and nervousness, anxiety, irritability, constipation, goiter, lack of sex-desire, ovary and testicles.

Loc : About 1/4 AI from little finger side edge on inner wrist fold adjoining the palm.

Relief Point # 115

Use : For bed wetting.

Loc : Two points, one on each of the two joints (inner and lower side) of little finger.

Relief Point # 116

Use : For pedotic (children's) pot belly.

Loc : Eight points, one point in center of middle joint (inner side) of each of four fingers of each hand.

RELIEF POINTS ON CHEST AND ABDOMEN

Relief Points on Chest & Abdomen

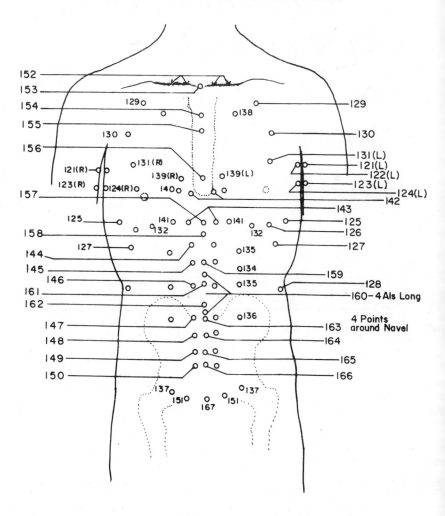

FIG. 4

4.5
RELIEF POINTS ON CHEST AND ABDOMEN

(Refer Fig. 4)

Relief Points # 121 (L) & (R)

    Use : Left point (L) for improvement of arterial blood circulation through the aorta, heart and body.
            Right point (R) for improvement of venous blood circulation through portal and liver.

    Loc : Two points, each being the highest point inside the arm pit and on the inner surface of arm, about 2 AIs above and 2-1/2 AIs outward from the nipple.

Relief Point # 122 (L) & (R)

    Use : Left - for left breast, the aorta, energy, lymph and arterial congestion against the left side of heart.

Right - for right breast and all the veins, used with RP # 34 in case of shock.

Loc : Both points in the arm pits on breast side and just opposite to RP # 121.

Relief Point # 123 (L) & (R)

Use : Left - for stomach disorders and emotions.

Loc : Under left arm pit and on the inner side of left arm at the level of left nipple.

Use : Right - for liver disorders.

Loc : Under the right arm pit and on the inner side of right arm at a level of right nipple.

Relief Point # 124

Use : For the whole reproductive system of both males and females, and emotions, ovaries and tubes.

Loc : Two points, each just in front of point 123 left and right on the outer edge of breasts.

Relief Point # 125 (L) and (R)

Use : Left - for breast and heart problems.
Right - for breast and liver problems.
Both for ribpains, poor lactation and face beauty

Loc : Under the outer and downward side of each breast, about 1 AI outward and 2 AIs below the nipples.

Relief Point # 126

Use : For rib pains and lack of milk in nursing mothers, lungs and bronchi.

Loc : Two points, one under each breast, 2.5 AIs from and vertically below each nipple.

Relief Point # 127
  Use : For gall bladder ailments.
  Loc : Two points, each about 4 AIs below and 1/2 AI outward from the nipple.

Relief Point # 128
  Use : For pain in abdomen, vomiting and arthritis (general, whole body).
  Loc : Two points, each on the side of body and below the arm pit, 2 AIs above and 5-1/2 AIs outer side of the navel.

Relief Point # 129
  Use : For common cold, cough and asthma.
  Loc : Two points, each between second and third rib, 4-1/2 AIs from central line of chest and 1-1/2 AIs below the notch at the throat base.

Relief Point # 130
  Use : For tetanus, tobacco poisoning, arterial circulation in lungs, intestines and colon.
  Loc : Two points, each 4 AIs above and 1/2 AI outer of nipple.

Relief Point # 131 (L) and (R)
  Use : Left - for arteries to colon, intestines and heart.
  Right - for veins from colon and intestines.
  Loc : Two points, each 2 AIs directly above the nipples.

Relief Point # 132 (L) and (R)

Use : Left - for left kidney and left side of colon. Right - for treating the right kidney and right side of colon.

Loc : Two points, each point located under and against the under side of each breast on the ribs at about 2-1/2 AIs below and 1-1/2 AIs towards breast bone from nipple.

Relief Point # 133

Use : For indigestion, gastritis, Gall bladder pain and all types of urine retention, accumulation of serous, serum, lymph, etc. in body cavities, fast heart.

Loc : Two points each at the bottom of ribs, about 5 AIs above navel and 2-1/2 AIs either side of center line of chest beat.

Relief Point # 134

Use : Cold, indigestion, gastritis, stomachache and nausea.

Loc : About 3.5 AIs navel and 2.5 AIs either side of center line of chest.

Relief Point # 135

Use : For constipation, gas.

Loc : Two points, each about 2.5 AIs above the naval and 2.5 AIs either side of center line.

Relief Point # 136

Use : For indigestion, colitis, diarrhoea.

Relief Points on Chest and Abdomen

Loc : Two points, each about 2-1/2 AIs either side and at the level of naval.

Relief Point # 137

Use : For lack of circulation from the legs and feet to the heart. In dilation of blood/lymph vessels and other problems of feet.

Loc : Two points, each on the crease of lower abdomen and thigh in the beginning of pubic cone, about 5 AIs below and 2-1/2 AIs either side of navel.

Relief Point # 138

Use : For back pains, lungs and bronchi.

Loc : Two points each about 2.5 AIs from central line of chest and 5 AIs above the nipple line.

Relief Point # 139 (L) and (R)

Use : Left - for mucous in bronchi, intestine and colon, heart and nerves.
Right - for constipation, gall bladder, heart, nerves and pancreas.

Loc : Two points, each is about 1-1/1 AIs above and 3 AIs towards center line of breast bone from each nipple.

Relief Point # 140 (L) and (R)

Use : Left - for breast, abdomen, rectum and anus, digestion problems, heart burn, gas, nausea and acid-indigestion.
Right - for breast, liver and ears.

Loc : Two points, at nipple level and 1-1/2 AIs either side of chest central line.

Relief Point # 141
- **Use :** For hormones to the heart.
- **Loc :** Two points, each 2 AIs from central chest line and 2 AIs below nipples, level.

Relief Point # 142
- **Use :** For cold, cough and asthma.
- **Loc :** Two points, each at 1 AI away from chest line and at level of nipples.

Relief Point # 143 (L) and (R)
- **Use :** Left – for spleen, anaemia and voice problems.
  Right – for pancreas, both points affect the hormones of the heart.
- **Loc :** Two points, each about 2 AIs below the nipples and 1.2 AIs either side of central line of chest.

Relief Point # 144
- **Use :** For stomachache.
- **Loc :** Two points, each about 5.2 AIs above naval and 1 AI either side of central line of stomach.

Relief Point # 145
- **Use :** For stomachache.
- **Loc :** Two points, each about 4 AIs above naval and 1 AI either side of central line of stomach.

Relief Point # 146 (L) and (R)
- **Use :** Right – for digestion and stimulation of food, intestines.

Left – for heart, intestines, constipation and cough patients.

Loc : Two points, each about 1 AI either side of central line through naval and 2 AIs above the naval.

Relief Point # 147

Use : For diarrhoea, abdomen pain.

Loc : Two points, each at the level of naval and 1 AI either side of it.

Relief point # 148

Use : For hip pain.

Loc : Two points – 1 AI below and 1 AI either side of navel.

Relief Point # 149 (R) and (L)

Use : Right – for colon disorders, gas, indigestion and appendicitis, sugar control.
Left – for colon disorders and constipation.

Loc : Two points, each about 2-1/2 AIs below navel and 1 AI either side central line through navel.

Relief Point # 150

Use : For hip pain, nausea, constipation, high blood pressure.

Loc : Two points, each about 3.5 AIs below navel and 1 AI either side of the central line.

Relief Point # 151

Use : For ovaries and tubes in the females and the spermatic cords in males. Pain in the legs and lower back, inability to walk and other difficulties during menopause.

Loc : Two points, each located in the center of pubic cone, 6 AIs below navel and 1-1/2 AIs away from central line.

Relief Point # 152

Use : Very important for all chemical changes for digestive system.

Loc : Upper margin of both collar bones, almost their half lengths from their center towards shoulders.

Relief Point # 153

Use : For treating esophagus, top valve of stomach, abdominal organs, kidneys, uterus, hernia, back and front of throat, cough, dyspnoea, asthma, hic-cough.

Loc : It is like a portion of cup at the upper margin of breast bone about 1 AI in length. Press or stimulate very softly without pressing deep in the notch.

Relief Point # 154

Use : For small intestines, abdominal bloat, water retention and dropsy, swelling of ankles and legs, thymus gland, ribs and bladder.

Loc : One point only, on the upper front center of the breast bone, about 5 AIs above nipples, line.

Relief Point # 155

Use : Acid indigestion, heart burn, cough, hic-cough, asthma, diphtheria.

Loc : One point only, about 1 AI below Relief Point # 154 or just below the bony ledge across the breast bone.

Relief Point # 156

- **Use :** For asthma, high blood pressure, lack of milk in nursing women and right side of heart.
- **Loc :** One point only, just in the middle of breast bone, 1/2 AI above the level of nipples. Press or massage with up and down motions of thumb.

Relief Point # 157

- **Use :** For obstruction for blood returning to heart through the great veins.
- **Loc :** One point only, just on the lowest tip of breast bone and 6-1/2 AIs above navel.

Relief Point # 158

- **Use :** For solar plexus, intestines, indigestion including stomach cramps, fainting and other mental disturbances, painful breathing.
- **Loc :** One point only, about 1 AI below the lowest tip of breast bone and 6 AIs above navel.

Relief Point # 159

- **Use :** For nausea, vomiting, diarrhoea, motion sickness, abdominal pain.
- **Loc :** One point only, in the middle of abdomen, about 4 AIs above the navel, midway between navel and the pit of stomach or solar plexus. Use thumb or palm to press or massage inward.

Relief Point # 160

- **Use :** For depression, loss of interest in life, feeling of suffocation, lump in throat, shivering, perspiration, excitement and despair, fatigue, memory deterioration, etc.

Loc : Portion of stomach between navel and back of ribs along the mid-line, about 4AIs in length upward from navel.

Relief Point # 161

Use : Abdomen pains, diarrhoea, high blood pressure, gastritis and nausea.

Loc : One point only about 2-1/2 AIs directly above navel and on central line.

Relief Point # 162

Use : Solar plexus, incontinence and retention of urine, bed wetting, worries, body energy and shock.

Loc : One point only at 1AI above navel directly above it.

Relief Point # 163

Use : For all digestive problems – gas, indigestion, duodenal ulcer, utilization of Calcium, oils, fat, sugar, starch, heart cases, chronic back pain and mental problems. Each point treats duodenum, points 3 and 4 on the left side, also treat the abdominal aorta. For gall bladder and bile ducts, press Relief Points # 143 (R) and # 139 (R) also.

```
              2       3    Left
     Right  (           )  Side
     Side   (  NAVEL    )
            (           )
              1       4

              4 POINTS
```

Loc : Four points around navel.

Relief Point # 164

Use : For abdominal swelling, disorders of bone-marrow of large hip-bones, hip-pains, lungs, congestion of left lung, cough, heart imbalance and dizziness, stomach ache, wet dreams, menstrual difficulties/irregularities, constipation, diarrhoea, prostate, etc.

Loc : One point only 1 AI directly below navel.

Relief Point # 165

Use : For stomach/abdominal pains, cramps, diarrhoea, wet dreams, menstrual pain and irregularities, constipation, hip-pain, frigidity and impotency, fatigue and urinary problems.

Loc : One point only 2-1/2 AIs directly below navel.

Relief Point # 166

Use : For wet dreams, frigidity, impotency, menstrual irregularities, cystitis.

Loc : One point only 3 AIs directly below navel.

Relief Point # 167

Use : For prostate, uterus and neck.

Loc : One point only, exactly in the middle where two pubic bones meet, about 6-1/2 AIs directly below navel.

Relief point # 168

Use : For water retention, treats ureter and bladder.

Loc : One point only, adjacent to RP # 167. It is contacted with finger if pressed straight in backward direction.

RELIEF POINTS ON BACK

Relief Points on Back

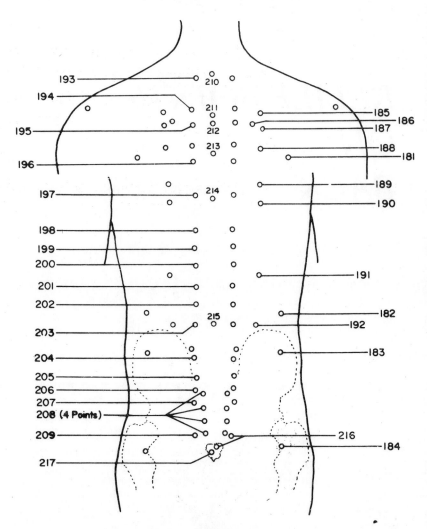

FIG. 5

4.6

RELIEF POINTS ON BACK

(Refer Fig. 5)

Note : *Distances of almost all relief points have been referred to the central line on spinal chord and its knob at the back of neck.*

Relief Point # 181

    Use : For shoulder pain, neuralgia, asthma, hand pain, elbow pain, bursitis. If necessary, treat with point # 152.

    Loc : Two points, each 6 AIs below and 5.5 AIs either side of spine knob on neck.

Relief Point # 182

    Use : For stomach ache, digestion, vomiting and abdominal pain.

    Loc : Two points, each 16-1/2 AIs below and 5 AIs either side of spine knob on neck.

Relief Point # 183

Use : For digestion, lower backache, sexual strength.

Loc : Two points, each 19 AIs below and 5 AIs either of spine knob on the neck.

Relief Point # 184

Use : For sciatica, lower backache, hip pain, colon trouble, lumbar pain, legs pain, sprain/strain at any place in the body, particularly for hip bone and intestine, all constipation cases, abdominal pain, infection, body shape-up.

Loc : Two points, each on the large indentation of hip at thigh bone, 25 AIs below and 5 AIs either side of spine knob on neck.

Relief Point # 185

Use : For Dowager's hump (curved by age).

Loc : Two points, each 2.5 AIs below and 3.5 AIs either side of spine knob on neck, between 3rd and 4th thoracic vertebrae.

Relief Point # 186

Use : For shoulder pain and whiplash.

Loc : Two points, each 3 AIs below and 3 AIs either side of spine knob at neck, between 3rd and 4th thoracic vertebrae.

Relief Point # 187

Use : for cough, neck and shoulder pain, panting.

Loc : Two points, each 3.5 AIs below and 3.5 AIs, either side of spine knob on neck, between 3rd and 4th thoracic vertebrae.

Relief Point # 188

Relief Points on Back

> Use : For poor circulation, asthma, shoulder pain, impotency and premature ejaculation, heart, lungs and flu.
>
> Loc : Two points, each 5 AIs below and 3-1/2 AIs either side of spine knob on neck, between 4th and 5th thoracic vertebrae and shoulder blade.

Relief Point # 189

> Use : For fevers, sweating, cough and asthma.
>
> Loc : Two points, each 7-1/2 AIs below and 3-1/2 AIs either side of spine knob on neck, between 6th and 7th thoracic vertebrae.

Relief Point # 190

> Use : For nausea, vomiting, hic-cup, gastritis.
>
> Loc : Two points, each 8-3/4 AIs below and 3-1/4 AIs either side of spine knob on neck, between 7th and 8th thoracic vertebrae.

Relief Point # 191

> Use : Diarrhoea, stomach ache, tension, nervous trouble, heart cases, difficult breathing, vital for life of cells all over the body, leg and hip pain.
>
> Loc : Two points, each 14 AIs below and 3 AIs either side of spine knob on neck, between 11th and 12th thoracic vertebrae.

Relief Point # 192

> Use : Lower backache, exhaustion, sexual strength, low energy, kidney trouble.
>
> Loc : Two points, each 17 AIs below and 3 AIs either side of spine knob on neck, between 2nd and 3rd lumbar vertebrae.

Relief Point # 193

Use : For headache, influenza, panting and high blood pressure.

Loc : Two points, each at 1-1/2 AIs on either side of spine knob on neck, between 7th cervical and 1st thoracic vertebrae. Use thumb to press hard towards the disc.

Relief Point # 194

Use : For common cold, cough, painful breathing, asthma, nasal obstructions, tension, congestion in neck and brain, mental fatigue, alcoholic effect, insomnia, every day tension and diabetes.

Loc : Two points, each 2-3/4 AIs below and 1-1/2 AIs either side of spine knob on neck, between 2nd and 3rd thoracic vertebrae.

Relief Point # 195

Use : Cough, painful/rapid breathing, asthma, headache, cold, spastic condition of arms, legs and hips, rashes such as measles, allergic diseases, hic-cough.

Loc : Two points, each 3-1/2 AIs below and 1-1/2 AIs either side of spine knob on neck, between 3rd and 4th thoracic vertebrae.

Relief Point # 196

Use : Irritability, weak heart, mental tension and anxiety.

Loc : Two points, each 6 AIs below and 1-1/2 AIs either side of spine knob on neck, between 5th and 6th thoracic vertebrae.

Relief Points on Back

Relief Point # 197

Use : For stomach ache, hic-cups, pains along ribs, asthma, cough, gastritis.

Loc : Two points, each 8-1/4 AIs below 1-1/2 AIs either side of spine knob on neck, between 7th and 8th thoracic vertebrae.

Relief Point # 198

Use : For pain along ribs, dizziness, sea/motion sickness, constipation, liver associated problems.

Loc : Two points, each 11 AIs below and 1-1/2 AIs either side of spine knob on neck, between 9th and 10th thoracic vertebrae.

Relief Point # 199

Use : For pain along ribs, dry mouth, gall-bladder problems, nausea.

Loc : Two points, each 12 AIs below and 1-1 AIs either side of spine knob on neck, between 10th and 11th thoracic vertebrae.

Relief Point # 200

Use : For diabetes, loss of appetite, spleen (pancreas) problems, nausea, gastritis, colitis.

Loc : Two points, each 13 AIs below and 1-1/2 AIs either side of spine knob on neck, between 11th and 12 th thoracic vertebrae.

Relief Point # 201 (L) and (R)

Use : Left – for stomach problems, gastritis, abdomen and thighs.
Right – for congestion and pain in gall bladder and appendix.

Both – for paralysis of legs, hypertension (H-B.P.).

Loc : Two points, each 15 AIs below and 1-1/2 AIs either side of spine knob on neck, between 12th thoracic and 1st lumbar vertebrae.

Relief Point # 202

Use : For diarrhoea, exhaustion, lower backache, poor blood circulation.

Loc : Two points, each 16 AIs below and 1-1/2 AIs either side of spine knob on neck, between 1st and 2nd lumbar vertebrae.

Relief Point # 203

Use : For body weakness, kidney associated problems, gall bladder, tension in abdomen and hip, leg pain, abdomen lymph, diabetes, frigidity, haemorrhoids, impotency, menopause, migraine, sexual stamina, ringing in the ears, headache, nasal obstruction, back ache, urinary problems, visual disturbances and glaucoma.

Loc : Two points, each 17-1/2 AIs below and 1-1/2 AIs either side of spine knob on neck, between 2nd and 3rd lumbar vertebrae.

Relief Point # 204

Use : For diarrhoea, constipation and problems of large intestine, cystitis.

Loc : Two points, each 19-1/2 AIs below and 1-1/2 AIs either side of spine knob on neck, between 4th and 5th lumbar vertebrae.

Relief Point # 205

Use : For lower back ache, digestion, sexual strength and impotency

Loc : Two points, each 21 AIs below and 1-1/2 AIs either side of spine knob on neck, between 5th lumbar vertebra and pelvic bone.

Relief Point # 206

Use : For lower backache, hip pain, small intestines related problems, constipation.

Loc : Two points, each 22 AIs below, 1-1/2 AIs either side of spine knob on neck, at the level of 1st sacral foramen.

Relief Point # 207

Use : For bed wetting and bladder problems.

Loc : Two points, each 23 AIs below and 1-1/2 AIs either side of spine knob on neck, at the level of 2nd sacral foramen.

Relief Point # 208

Use : For nerves which affect the body from rectum to brain, back and reproductive organs.

Loc : Eight point or openings in the bone of sacrum each about 1 AI from central line and 1 AI from each other, all between RPs # 206 and 209.

Relief Point # 209

Use : For bed wetting, menstrual irregularities.

Loc : Two points, each 25 1/2 AIs below and 1-1/2 AIs either side of spine knob on neck, on the level of 4th groove of sacrum.

Relief Point # 210

Use : For fevers, cold, headaches, allergies, asthma, sinus, nose bleed, problems in pituitary, thyroid, spinal cord/nerve, and every bone in the body, swallowing difficulty, fatigue, heart problems. Very important point– cough and hic-cough.

Loc : One point only, at the spine knob on neck between 7th cervical and 1st thoracic vertebral. More visible on neck when head is bent forward to touch the chest with chin.

Relief Point # 211

Use : For cold, headache, influenza.

Loc : One point, only 3 AIs directly below spine knob on the neck.

Relief Point # 212

Use : For cold, asthma.

Loc : One point only, 3-1/2 AIs directly below spine knob on the neck.

Relief Point # 213

Use : For cold, sun or heat stroke.

Loc : One point only, 5-1/2 AIs directly below spine knob at neck.

Relief Point # 214

Use : For impotency.

Loc : One point only, 8-1/2 AIs directly below spine knob at the neck and almost between the two points of RP # 197.

Relief Point # 215

Use : For impotency, wet dreams, lumbar pain, headache, ringing in the ears.

Loc : One point only, 17-1/2 AIs directly below spine knob on the neck. Between 2nd and 3rd lumbar vertebrae just behind the navel and between the two points of RP # 203.

Relief Point # 216

Use : For reproductive organs, brain, stomach problems, constipation.

Loc : One point only, on the tip of a small bone (called tail bone) and towards anus. Press the tip towards head and hold for a minute.

Relief Point # 217

Use : For rectal pain.

Loc : A bony circle around and about 2 inches inside the anus on all sides, which can be contacted/pressed only by hooking a finger inside.

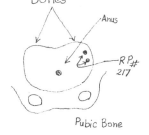

RELIEF POINTS ON LEGS

Relief Points on Legs

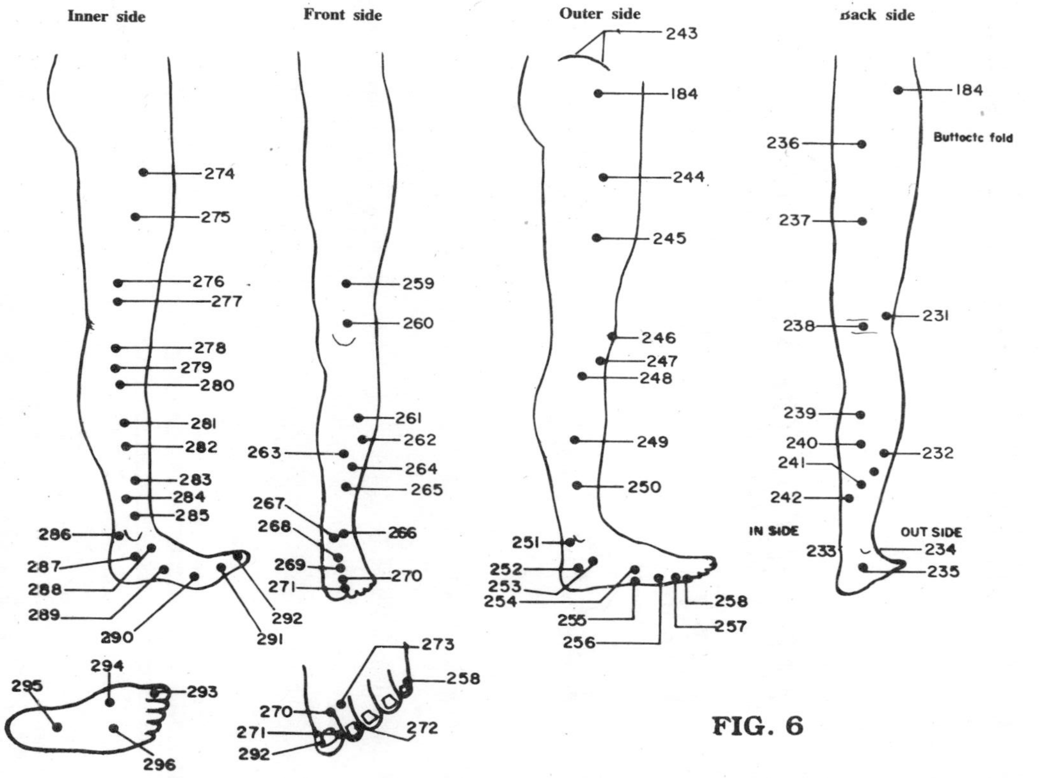

FIG. 6

4.7

RELIEF POINTS ON LEGS

(Refer Fig. 6)

Note : *One point is at similar location on each leg and has the same use. Both leg-points are to be treated simultaneously or alternately.*

A. Relief Points on Back Side of Leg:

Relief Point # 231

    Use : For constipation.

    Loc : 1 AI above the back knee fold and 1/2 AI from the outer edge.

Relief Point # 232

    Use : Excellent for leg and body muscles.

    Loc : About 9 AIs below the back knee fold and 1 AI from the outer edge.

Relief Point # 233 (Outside and inside)

    Use : Outside - For constipation or accumulation

of blood vessels.
Inside – For energy to body tissues.
Both – For constrictions and foot trouble.

Loc : Around both ankle bones – outside and inside of a foot. For better results, press the ankle bone from around and outside the edge towards inside and against the bone.

Relief Point # 234

Use : For swelling and pain of twisted ankle.

Loc : Two points just below both inner and outer ankle bones.

Relief Point # 235

Use : For mucus passage from lungs to the intestine, constipation and hip pain. Use relief point # 139 left also.

Loc : Mid-way between the ankle bone and the lowest point on the heel.

Relief Point # 236

Use : For sciatica, lower backache that travels into buttock, hip pain, arthritis and constipation.

Loc : At the base of hip at thigh bone and at the line of buttock fold, about one fourth of its width from inner edge.

Relief Point # 237

Use : For sciatica, tired legs and leg pain.

Loc : 5-1/2 Als below buttock fold and 1 Al towards inner side from the middle of back of thigh, 7-1/2 Als above inner knee fold.

Relief Points on Legs

Relief Point # 238

Use : Sciatica, lower backache, calf spasm, lumbago, rashes/infectious diseases such as measles, constitutional and allergies such as eczema, hives with red, painful velvety swelling. Pain in thigh, knee and calf.

Loc : At the center of fold at the back of knee (knee-back fold).

Relief Point # 239

Use : For pain in center of calf muscles, leg pain and colon problems. Sciatica which travels down the leg.

Loc : In the center of the heavy calf muscles at the back of leg, 9 AIs above ankles.

Relief Point # 240

Use : For sciatica, spasm of muscles, tired legs, back and calf pain, cramp and paralysis of legs.

Loc : 7 AIs above the inner ankle bone, exactly in the hollow in the lower middle portion of calf, almost half way between inner knee fold and top of heal.

Relief Point # 241

Use : Excellent for rheumatic arthritis, foot pain.

Loc : 4 AIs above inner ankle bone and 1 AI inside edge.

Relief Point # 242

Use : For ankle pain, diarrhoea, cough, cold, insomnia and sciatica.

Loc : On the lower leg 3 AIs above the inner ankle bone and on inner edge of the leg.

B. Relief Points on Outer Side of Legs:-

Relief Point # 243

  Use : For problems of intestines, indigestion, amino acids and obesity, use with RP # 184 if weight gain is a problem.

  Loc : About 3 AIs long along the top crest of hip bones. Press with your thumbs on both hip bones at the same time.

Relief Point # 244

  Use : For colon problems.

  Loc : Close to the crease at the junction of thigh and trunk, about 6 AIs below RP # 184 on the outer side of thigh bone and 11 AIs above knee fold.

Relief Point # 245

  Use : For circulation in legs, tired legs.

  Loc : On the outer side of thigh and at the tip of the middle finger when the arms are held straight down, about 6 AIs above the knee.

Relief Point # 246

  Use : For fevers and paralysis of legs, Hip pain, arthritis, knee pain and insomnia.

  Loc : Four points two on each Leg one in each depression just below knee cap either side of the bone.

Relief Point # 247

  Use : Works as a tonic for elderly people, leg muscles, burning sensation, diabetes, eye problems, abdominal lymph and bloat, thyroid, obesity, headache, vomiting, dizziness, deafness, cough, constipation.

Loc : About 2-1/2 AIs below and outer side of knee cap bottom.

Relief Point # 248

Use : For knee and ankle pain, gall-bladder pain, diarrhoea and cholera, frigidity and infertility, fatigue, headache, migraine, urinary problems, paralysis of legs.

Loc : About 4 AIs below knee cap, center and outer side of leg.

Relief Point # 249

Use : For arthritis general, hip and leg pains, tired legs, reproductive hormones, tension, gall-bladder pain.

Loc : About 8 AIs below knee cap, center and outer side of leg, just behind long thin bone and hal-fway between ankle and knee.

Relief Point # 250

Use : For legs/ankle pain and sciatica, pain due to over eating, drinking, body shape-up.

Loc : About 4 AIs above outer ankle bone and in the middle of outer surface.

Relief Point # 251

Use : For snake bite, sciatica, dizziness, epilepsy, general neuralgia, lumbar pain, hip pain; general arthritis, leg, ankle and back pains/sprains, foot ailments/ injuries, oedema and arthritis.

Loc : In the depression just in back/behind the outer ankle bone. Use thumb to press hard.

Relief Point # 252

Use : For foot pain, lumbago, neuralgia, pains in abdomen and colon.

Loc : In the depression immediately below outer ankle and 1-1/2 AIs above heel bottom.

Relief Point # 253

Use : For gall-bladder problems.

Loc : On the outer surface immediately in front and slightly below the outer ankle bone.

Relief Point # 254

Use : For menstrual irregularities, ringing in the ears and foot pain.

Loc : In the depression between 4th and 5th toes, 2-1/2 AIs up from the bridge between these toes and 1AI from side edge and above the bump.

Relief Point # 255

Use : For nasal obstruction, neck pain, stiff neck, bee sting.

Loc : On the outer edge just in the side and under the bump, about 2-1/2 AIs from little toe knuckle along the outer edge.

Relief Point # 256

Use : For bee sting, burns and scalds, insect bites, sunburn, wound and cuts.

Loc : On the outer edge of foot in the depression I

AI behind of little toe knuckle and 1-1/2 AIs forward of RP # 255.

Relief Point # 257
- **Use :** For nasal obstruction, neck pain.
- **Loc :** On the outer edge of foot and just in front of little toe knuckle.

Relief Point # 258
- **Use :** For intestinal worms, fungal infection of skin, neck pain, nasal obstruction, difficult labour.
- **Loc :** At the end of little toe at the intersection of two lines – one along base and the other along outer side of the nail.

C. *Relief Points on Front side of Legs:-*

Relief Point # 259
- **Use :** For stomachache /cramps, arthritis in the knee, diarrhoea, breast pain, ankle/foot ailment/injuries, oedema and arthritis.
- **Loc :** 3 AIs above the top of knee cap and slightly outer side from center of leg width.

Relief Point # 260
- **Use :** For malfunction of knee and heart.
- **Loc :** Just at the top of knee cap.

Relief Point # 261
- **Use :** For colitis, gastritis, diarrhoea, rheumatoid arthritis and stomachache.
- **Loc :** 6-1/2 AIs below knee cap along the outer edge of central bone.

Relief Point # 262
>   **Use :** For lumbago, leg pain.
>   **Loc :** 8 AIs below knee cap and on outer edge of central bone. Almost middle of the distance between knee cap and ankles.

Relief Point # 263
>   **Use :** For problems of colon.
>   **Loc :** About 9 AIs below the knee and on the middle of leg front.

Relief Point # 264
>   **Use :** For colitis.
>   **Loc :** 10 AIs below knee cap and on outer edge of central bone.

Relief Point # 265
>   **Use :** For pains due to over-eating, over drinking, headache.
>   **Loc :** About 4 AIs above the ankle level and in middle of leg front.

Relief Point # 266
>   **Use :** For all problems of eyes of their muscles.
>   **Loc :** Just on the outside of stringy muscles at the top of the foot.

Relief Point # 267
>   **Use :** Arthritis of ankle, lower backache, high blood pressure.
>   **Loc :** In the shallow space between front of inner ankle bone and stringy muscles at the top of

Relief Points on Legs 111

the foot, and about 0.8 AI from RP # 266. Thus the two RPs # 266 and # 267 are on either side of foot top muscles.

Relief Point # 268

    Use : For headache and dizziness, muscle cramp, ringing in ears, deafness.

    Loc : 1-1/2 AIs up from the toe knuckle on upper surface of foot between 1st and 2nd toes.

Relief Point # 269

    Use : For headache and dizziness, suffocation, swelling (oedema), muscle cramp.

    Loc : 1 AI up from the toe knuckle between 1st and 2nd toes and at the junction of their bones.

Relief Point # 270

    Use : For muscle cramps, pain or tension in ureters and bladder. For kidney stones, use with RP # 132, also for kidney.

    Loc : At the web between the big toe and the adjacent (second) toe.

Relief Point # 271

    Use : For relieving constipation, diarrhoea.

    Loc : At the inside corner of nail of big toe.

Relief Point # 272

    Use : For insomnia – sleeplessness, wounds, cuts.

    Loc : At the corner of the nail of 2nd toe near to the 3rd toe.

Relief Point # 273

    Use : For pains in foot or toes.

    Loc : At the base of the second toe and near third toe.

D. Relief Points on Inner Side of Legs:-

Relief Point # 274

    Use : For insomnia, low blood pressure and menstrual pains.

    Loc : 10 AIs above knee and 2 AIs from front surface of thigh.

Relief Point # 275

    Use : For frigidity and sexual vigour, menstrual pains, low blood pressure, insomnia.

    Loc : 7.6 AIs above knee on upper thigh and about $2\frac{1}{2}$ from front surface of the thigh.

Relief Point # 276

    Use : For menstrual pains and irregularities, cystitis, hives, itching, neuro-dermatitis, obesity.

    Loc : 3 AIs above the knee cap center and almost middle of the inner surface.

Relief Point # 277

    Use : For itching, allergic eczema, hives, menstrual pains and irregularities, neuro-dermatitis, intestinal problems.

    Loc : About 1-1/2 AIs above knee and at the center of thigh – inner face of leg.

Relief Point # 278

Use : For pains in knee, abdomen, intestines, and spleen. Also for dizziness, constipation, diarrhoea, paralysis of leg, menstrual irregularities.

Loc : In the center of inner side of lower leg, 1-1/2 AIs below knee level and in a small depression just below the bone.

Relief Point # 279

Use : For abdominal pain, cystitis, frigidity and infertility, wound and cuts.

Loc : 2 AIs below inner knee fold and at the center of inner surface of leg.

Relief Point # 280

Use : For sexual vigour, frigidity, arthritis, menstrual irregularities.

Loc : 4 AIs below knee fold at the center of inner surface.

Relief Point # 281

Use : For nausea, frigidity, confused mental thinking, pituitary, drugs addiction.

Loc : 7 AIs below knee fold slightly toward sfront edge.

Relief Point # 282

Use : For leg pain, ankle pain.

Loc : 8-1/2 AIs below knee fold and at the middle of inner surface.

Relief Point # 283

    Use : For frigidity.

    Loc : 4 AIs above inner ankle bone slightly towards front side edge.

Relief Point # 284

    Use : For injury like pain in ankle, sciatica, over-weight, insomnia, digestive problems, any female sexual problem, cold, cough, leg pain, menstrual cramps, irregularities and pain, nasal obstruction, frigidity, impotency, premature ejaculation; spleen, liver and kidney meridians are stimulated by this point. Helps in easy and smooth child delivery, abdomen pain, urinary problems, oedema and arthritis, foot ailments, diarrhoea.

    Loc : 3 AIs above inner ankle bone, slightly towards back side edge.

Relief Point # 285

    Use : For gastritis, constipation, diarrhoea, abdominal pain, cholera, motion sickness, nausea, insomnia, sexual vigour, impotency, difficult labour, problems of sex, headache, cold, hic-cups, tiredness and pain in legs.

    Loc : 1-1/2 AIs above inner ankle bone, slightly towards backside edge.

Relief Point # 286

    Use : For suffocation, cough, back/leg/ankle and foot pain, fatigue, body pain, tension in neck and shoulders, urinary problems, oedema and arthritis.

Relief Points on Legs

Loc : In the depression just in the back/behind of inner ankle bone. It is just opposite to RP # 251 which is behind the outer ankle bone.

Relief Point # 287

Use : For haemorrhage, concussion, bee sting, frost bite, snake bite, kidney malfunction.

Loc : In the hollow space just below inner ankle bone just opposite to RP # 252 located below the outer ankle bone.

Relief Point # 288

Use : For indigestion, constipation, ankle injuries, oedema and arthritis, foot ailments.

Loc : In the depression just in front and slightly below the inner ankle bone and just opposite to RP # 253 which is located in front and slightly below the outer ankle bone.

Relief Point # 289

Use : For painful breathing, air swallowing (aerophagia), heart burn and chest pain, stomach ulcers and problems of gall stone, spleen and pancreas.

Loc : On the inner lower edge of foot about 1/2 AI above the sole just above the depression of sole. The point is almost 4 AIs from rear end of heel and 6 AIs from front end of big toe.

Relief Point # 290

Use : For nausea, testicle injury or pain, menstrual irregularities, insomnia.

Loc : On the inner edge of foot 1 AI back from big toe joint behind the bony protrusion.

Relief Point # 291

Use : For indigestion, nausea, exhaustion.

Loc : Outside the big toe and just in front of its knuckle.

Relief Point # 292

Use : For regulating long periods, heavy bleeding and other menstrual irregularities.

Loc : On the big toe nail where lines along the base and outer side of nail intersect.

E. Relief Points at the Sole of Foot :-

Relief Point # 293

Use : For difficult breathing, flu, problems with pituitary and lungs. Press hard with thumb.

Loc : At the center of the bottom of the big toe.

Relief Point # 294

Use : For pain in bunions, prostate and reproductive organs, gout.

Loc : At the rear of the prominent joint at the base of the big toe.

Relief Point # 295

Use : For energy to brain. Important for inflammatory conditions such as colitis.

Loc : In the center of the bottom of the foot just in front of the heel prominence.

Relief Point # 296

Use : For fainting, shock, sun/heat stroke, suffocation, syncope, menstrual pain. Gives energy to the weak body.

Loc : In the depression on the bottom of the foot, just in the back of the ball, when the foot is raised. About one-third from tip of third toe and two-third from rear of the heel. Press hard to activate.

ACUPRESSURE FOR MAINTAINING GOOD HEALTH

5.

ACUPRESSURE FOR MAINTAINING GOOD HEALTH

A. STEPS FOR MAINTAINING HEALTHY BODY :-

1. **Warming-up :**
    (a) Rubbing the palms with each other, very fast and forcefully.
    (b) Every time, when the palms are warm enough by rubbing, touch them on your face on the left cheek, move to forehead and then move to the right cheek. Next time reverse the direction. Do so for six times and seventh, the last time, making cups of your palms, put them on your eyes (closed) and continue for a minute thinking that you are in a totally dark place or covered with a black cloth. It will soothe your eyes.

2. **Massage your Head :**
    (a) Massage or press the three Relief Points with the tips of your middle fingers, RPs # 5 and # 11 on head and RP # 210 on top of back in

succession for about a minute.

(b) Hold your head placing the surface of RP # 106 of your palms on each temple (a portion of head between eye and ear) and push from front hair line to back hair-line on the nape. Do it for seven times.

3. **Wiping the Forehead:**

Wipe your forehead seven times slowly with the tips of your both hands fingers from the middle of the eyebrows to front hair line above and then move to both sides.

4. **Stimulate the Ears:**

(a) Place your palms over your ears and fingers of each hand at the back of the skull. Then vibrate the palms with a set frequency against both ears for 21 times.

(b) Placing the palms and fingers as in 4 (a), knock the back of skull with index and middle finger bilaterally so that a sound like "DONG" is clearly heard for 21 times.

5. **Massaging the Eyes:**

(a) With the knuckles of your fingers, massage gently the sockets of the two eyes for seven times from their inner side to the upper and outer side and then from outer to upper and inner side keeping the eyes closed.

(b) Use the tips of your fingers or thumbs to massage gently the relief points # 25, # 24, # 26 and # 27, repeating each process for seven times keeping the eyes closed.

6. **Massaging the Mouth Inside:**

   Sweep the space between the teeth and lips with your tongue up and down clockwise and anti-clockwise seven times each.

7. **Knocking the Lips and Teeth:**

   Close your mouth lightly and knock the upper and lower lips/teeth clock and anti-clockwise in seven rounds.

8. **Slapping the Chin:**

   Slap the under side of your chin with the fingers of each hand alternately (keeping palms down-ward) rhythmically for about 21 times.

9. **Massaging Shoulders:**

   Massage both points RP # 61 on your shoulders simultaneously or alternately with your thumbs for a minute.

10. **Slapping the Chest:**

    Slap your chest with the fingers of both hands rhythmically while breathing deeply for about 21 times.

11. **Massaging the Flanks:**

    Using the area around RP # 106 at your hands, massage both the flanks (sides between last rib and the hip) rapidly for 21 times each side.

12. **Massaging the Abdomen:**

    Place RP # 114 of your one hand on your navel and place the other hand over it for more pressure, then push both hands with force in a clockwise direction for 21 times. Now change the hands one over the other and repeat the exercise again 21 times.

13. **Massaging the Back:**

Rub the sides of the back upwards and downwards with knuckles of each hand (holding both hands as fists) forcefully for 5 minutes.

14. **Massaging the Spine and Sacrum:**

Make fists of your both hands and hit both sides at 1-1/2 AIs of your spine moving the hands from down to upwards while hitting between sacrum and shoulders. Make up and down seven rounds.

15. **Massaging Thighs:**

Massage your thighs with your palms forcefully from down to upwards about 21 times.

16. **Massaging Knee:**

Massage the area around knee, particularly RP # 247, for a minute.

17. **Gripping the Calves:**

Grip the calf muscles firmly with fingers down from heel to up the calf, first the left leg and then the right one, each for about 21 times. Massage RPs # 249 and # 284 also 21 times or 1 minute each.

18. **Massaging Hands and Feet:**

Massage RPs # 76, # 111 and # 114 at the hands; RPs # 291 and # 294 at the feet with your thumb for a minute or 21 times each.

Depending up on the circumstances, it is better to do all the above 18 points in the morning. If, any how, it is not convenient to do all at a time, then do the first 12 in the morning before breakfast and the remaining 6 (i.e. 13 to 18) in the night before going to bed but at least 3 hours after food.

B. STEPS FOR MAINTAINING HEALTHY EYES:-

For maintaining healthy eyes, the following exercises should be carried out once after a prolonged use of eyes (for example continuous reading or doing fine needle work etc.), otherwise once in the morning or evening.

1. **Washing and Warming-up of Hands and Eyes:**

Before carrying out the actual exercises, wash your hands with soap and eyes with cold water sprinkling it on eyes when a handful of cold water is filled in the mouth also. Make them dry with soft warm towel. Rub the palms together rapidly to warm them and put the warm palms on the eyes. Do so seven times.

2. **Wiping the Forehead:**

Wipe your forehead 7 times slowly with the tips of fingers of your both hands from the middle of the eyebrows to front hair line above upto RP # 16 and then both sides, massage RPs # 18, # 19 and # 20 also.

3. **Massaging the Upper Orbits:**

Close your eyes, put the four fingers of each hand on the forehead and ball of thumbs upon the upper orbit of each eye beneath the eye-brows and massage softly RPs # 24 and # 26 carefully when the eyes are closed.

4. **Massaging the Nose-root:**

Close the eyes and massage RP # 25, ends of nose-root upwards with the thumb-ball and downwards with the ball of index finger. Repeat this procedure for about 21 times.

5. **Massaging the Cheeks:**

Place your thumb at the depression of RP # 41

below lower jaw and index finger on RP # 27 below the eyes and above the cheeks. Keeping the other fingers in the form of fists, massage the cheeks centrally and applying pressure from down to upward between RPs # 27 and # 41 with index finger balls for a minute or so.

PRECAUTIONS

6.

PRECAUTIONS

1. Do not start giving acupressure to a patient unless you have known him and his condition completely through consultation, physical examination, other tests and diagnosis. If it is known or suspected, the patient is seriously ill, don't give him acupressure. Better send him or her to the hospital.

2. Don't treat patients with contagious diseases such as measles, whooping cough, malaria, osteomyelitis or any disorders involving organs such as heart, liver, kidney, lung, or cancer, sarcoma, infectious diseases, broken bones, etc.

3. Beware, if patients is suspected to have internal bleeding, conditions such as ulcers, duodenal ulcers, haemophilia, etc. which can be triggered by external forces.

4. Don't treat when your patient is very hungry, or very full. After eating a big meal, wait at least for two hours. If very hungry, wait until he has eaten a little.

5. If the patient is very tired, sweating heavily, or has a fast heartbeat, wait until he gets normal.

6. Be sure that the patient is happy and relaxed. Don't treat patient just after bath, excretion, worry or other such work/thing.

7. Pregnant female patient should not be treated with acupressure unless her doctors have recommended otherwise.

8. Don't use sharp objects that could injure the skin. It should be of enough girth to apply pressure to a defined area on a nerve.

9. Points on/near the eyes are to be treated very gently and carefully with finger or thumb and when the eyes are closed.

10. Acupressure, by no means, be taken as a substitute for medical consultation, advice and supervision.

11. Alcoholic, very cold or hot drinks, irritating, sour & iced foods, etc. which may have adverse effects on the patient, should be avoided atleast during treatment period. It is always better to suggest some drinks and foods which may help the patient to recover early and to regain strength.

12. It is seen that some people for the sake of getting relief quickly, stimulate the relief point either more than the schedule period or more than two times in 24 hours or do both the things. Doing so in either way is wrong and harmful. It produces toxin and makes body weak.

7.

ABBREVIATIONS

AP = Acupressure
RP = Relief Point
AI = Acupressure-Inch
Pt = Patient
Pr = Practitioner
Loc = Location
Esp. = Especially

INDEX OF DISESES AND THEIR RELIEF POINTS

(Showing malfunctioning body parts/ailments and concerned relief points)

A

Abdominal
   aorta-163
   bloat-154, 247
   cramp-5
   lymph-203, 247
   organs-153
   pain-128, 140, 147, 159, 161, 182, 184, 2011, 203, 252, 278, 279, 284, 285
   soothed-17
   swelling-164
Abscess-1
Accumulation of
   blood-233 outer
   serous, serum & lymph-133
Aches
   ear-8, 76A
   eyes-25
   lower back-183, 184, 192, 202, 205, 206, 236, 267
   stomach-24, 36, 134, 144, 145, 164, 182, 191, 197, 261
   tooth-32, 33, 34, 35, 36, 41, 76A
   wrist/hand-84, 89.
Acid Indigestion-81, 140L, 155
Acne-34
Addiction drugs-7, 29, 281
Aerophagia - 74, 289
Ailment winter-16
Alcoholic effect-194
Allergic eczema-277
Allergic diseases-195
Allergy-13, 16, 30, 210, 238

Index of Diseases and their Relief Points

Amino Acids-243
Anaemia- 51, 143 L
Angina-74, 83
Ankle injuries-288
Ankle pain-76A, 234, 242, 250, 251, 259, 282, 284, 286
Ankle twisted-234
Anus-140 L
Anxiety-10, 23, 76 A, 87, 113, 114, 196
Apoplexy-64
Appendicitis-149 R
Appendix Pain-201 R
Appetite loss-8, 200
Arms
    pain-56 R, 65, 79
    fatigue-72
    tired-107
Arterial Circulation
    lungs-130
    intestines-130, 131 L
    colon-130, 131 L
    heart-131 L
Arterial Congestion-122 L
Arthritis
    general-63, 76A, 108B, 128, 236, 246, 248, 251, 280
    rheumatic-241, 261
    ankle-267
    knee-259
Asthma-54, 61, 101, 103, 129, 142, 153, 155, 156, 181, 188, 189, 193, 194, 195, 197, 200, 210, 212

B

Back pain-85, 138, 163, 203, 208, 240, 251, 286
Bags below eyes-27
Bed wetting-13, 115, 162, 207, 209
Bee Sting-255, 256, 287
Bile Ducts-163
Bite
    frost-287
    insect-256
    snake-112, 251, 287
Bladder-154, 168, 207
Bleeding Nose-1, 2, 4, 11, 12, 13, 29, 30, 76A, 107, 210
Blepharitis-24, 76A
Blood Circulation Improvement
    heart-34, 121 L, 122 L
    body muscle-34
    eyes-34
    aorta-121 L, 122 L
    body-121L
    portal-121R
    liver-121R
Blurred Vision-20
Body
    chemistry-18
    energy - 162
    general - 56

Index of Diseses and their Relief Points

muscles-232
pain-286
weakness-203
stiffness-101
shape-up-4, 11, 76A, 184, 250

Boil ear-8

Bone
general-210
marrow-164

Breast
right-122R, 125R, 140R,
left-122L, 125L
pain-85, 140, 259

Breathing
problems-22, 101, 104, 107, 112, 158, 191, 194, 293
short/rapid-195

Bronchi-126, 138

Bronchitis-104, 112

Bruises-64

Bunion pain-294

Burn
fire-256
sun-109, 256

Burning sensation-247

Bursitis-62, 71, 73, 80, 101, 112, 181

C

Calcium utilization-163

Calf spasm-238

Cataract-39

Chemical changes (in digesstion) - 152

Chemistry of body-18

Chest pain-74, 83, 103, 125, 289

Child delivery-284

Children's convulsions-43

Cholera-248, 285

Chronic infection - 16

Chyle-51

Circulation help
liver to heart-65
arms and hands-82
legs to heart-137, 244
poor-188, 202
artery to lungs-130
artery to intestines-130, 131 L
artery to colon-130, 131 L

Clot in lungs-83

Cold-2, 16, 30, 61, 76A, 84, 88, 134, 142, 195, 210, 211, 212, 213, 242, 284, 285

Colitis-136, 200, 261, 264, 295

Colon
left-132 L
right-132 R
both sides-149, 252, 263

Common cold-10, 11, 12, 13, 30, 54, 76A, 88, 103, 129, 194

Concussion-64, 109, 287

Confused Thinking-281

Congestion in
brain-194
gall bladder-201R
left heart-122L
left lung-164
neck-194
veins-8

Conjunctivitis 11, 22, 25, 30, 76A

Consciousness loss-31

Constant headache-247

Constipation-9, 79, 84, 113, 114, 135, 139R, 146L, 149L, 150, 164, 165, 184, 198 204, 206, 216, 231, 233, 235, 236, 247, 271, 278, 285, 288

Constitutional disease-238

Constriction blood vessels outer -233

Controls
body weight-55
temperature-55
sugar-88, 149R

Cough-54, 101, 102, 103, 104, 106, 107, 112, 129, 142, 146L, 153, 155, 164, 187, 189, 194, 195, 197, 210, 242, 247, 278, 284, 286

Cramps
abdomen-5
calf-240
stomach-158, 165, 250

Crow's feet-22, 26

Crushed tissue-64

Cuts-63, 256, 272, 279

Cystitis- 166, 204, 276, 279

D

Deafness-11, 15, 34, 76A, 247, 268

Deformed fingers-92

Depression-5, 110, 160

Dermatitis-276

Despair-5, 110, 160

Diabetes-194, 200, 203, 247

Diarrhoea-71, 76A, 79, 136, 147, 159, 161, 164, 165, 191, 202, 204, 242, 248, 259, 261, 271, 278, 284, 285

Digestion-74, 140L, 146R, 182, 183, 205, 283

Dilation of
blood vessels-137
lymph vessels-137
Diphtheria-155

Index of Diseses and their Relief Points

Disorders of
   bone marrow of large hip bones-164
   colon-14, 33, 149R & L
   ears-14
   intestine-14
   kidney-33
   liver-123R
   pituitary-18
   stomach-24, 123L

Dizziness-2, 11, 15, 21, 23, 31, 34, 164, 198, 247, 251, 268, 269, 278

Double vision-21

Dowager's hump-185

Dropsy-154

Drowsiness-42

Drug addiction-7, 29, 281

Dry eyes-26

Dry mouth-199

Duodenal ulcer-28, 163

Dyspnoea-153

E

Ear
   ache-8, 34, 76A
   disorder-14, 140R
   ringing in-33, 34, 203, 215
   vein-8
   wax-32, 76A.

Eczema-238

Elbow pain -63, 76A, 88, 101, 112, 181

Electric shock -29, 31, 109, 114

Emergency Points for
   dizziness-31
   epilepsy-31, 251
   fainting-31
   nausea-31

Emotions-123L, 124

Energize
   around eyes-24
   around mouth-38
   body-61
   brain-295
   below eyes-27
   body tissues inner-233
   low energy-192
   head and scalp-17, 54
   face-17, 19, 35, 38
   face muscles-19, 27, 52
   forehead-17
   jaw lock-35
   local muscl-52
   neck-19, 54
   skin-19
   throat/neck-52, 54
   weak body-296
   wholebody-52, 61, 122 L, 162

Epilepsy-31, 251

Excess fluid-6, 39

Excitement-110, 160

Exhaustion-64, 78, 111, 112, 192, 202, 291

Eyes
   ache-25
   beautification-22, 24, 30, 76A
   excess fluid-39
   irritation-16, 26
   problems-61, 247, 266
   red, swollen-11, 21, 24, 25, 76A
   soreness-16, 61
   strain-24, 27
   swollen-11

F

Face beauty-24, 125

Face energized-17, 21

Face rejuvenation-30, 125

Facial pain-27, 32, 35, 103

Facial tension-27, 30, 32, 76A

Fainting-31, 91, 114, 158, 160, 296

Fast heart-133

Fatigue-11, 61, 64, 110, 160, 165, 210, 248, 286

Fatigue of arms-72, 76A, 111.

Female sexual problems-284

Fever common-71, 189, 210, 246

hay-10, 16
rheumatic-77
cold-88
with lung problems-101

Fingers deformed/knocked, etc.-92

Flu-16, 188, 293

Foot pain-241, 251, 252, 254, 284, 286, 288

Foot trouble-133, 233 both

Foot ailment/injuries-251, 259, 284, 288

Forehead energy-17

Frigidity-52, 76A, 11, 165, 166, 203, 248, 275, 279, 280, 281, 283, 284

Frost bite-287

Frozen shoulders-62

Fungal infection-258

G

Gall bladder
   energy-17
   general-1, 127, 139R, 163, 199, 203
   pain-76A, 133, 201, 248, 249
   problem-253
   pus or abscess-1

Gall stone-74, 289

Gas-5, 9, 135, 140L, 149R, 163

Gas indigestion-9, 163

Index of Diseses and their Relief Points

Gastritis-134, 161, 190, 197, 200, 201L, 261, 285
Gingivitis-76A, 107, 134
Glaucoma-22, 24, 25, 39, 76A, 203
Goiter-24, 114
Gout-78, 294

H

Hand and wrist pain-89, 181
Hand spasm-107
Hay fever-10, 16, 76A
Head
  colds-15, 37, 76A
  injuries-64
  hurts-11
Headache-1, 2, 3, 4, 5, 6, 7, 11, 12, 13, 15, 17, 19, 21, 22, 23, 24, 26, 61, 71, 75, 76A, 90, 103, 104, 113, 193, 195, 203, 210, 211, 215, 248, 265, 268, 269, 285
Headache with pressure-3
Hearing loss-8
Heart
  attack-34, 83
  blood circulation-34, 157
  burn-74, 140L, 155, 289
  general-56, 125L, 139, 146L, 188, 191, 210
  imbalance-164
  irregular beat-114
  pain-83
  problems-5, 6, 163, 210, 260
  palpitation-55, 108B, 114
  right side-156
Heavy menstrual bleeding-292
Haemorrhage-13, 64, 112, 287
Haemorrhoids-5, 203
Hernia-153, 155
Hic-cough-76A, 86, 101, 103, 153, 155, 188, 195, 210
Hic-cups-190, 197, 285
High blood pressure-23, 24, 52, 71, 150, 156, 161, 193, 201, 210, 267
Hip bone strain-184
Hip bone marrow-164
Hip pain-148, 150, 164, 165, 184, 191, 206, 235, 236, 246, 249, 251
Hives-238, 276, 277
Hoarseness-54
Hormones to hearts-141, 143
Hypertension (H-B.P.)-24, 210

Hysteria-106

I

Imbalance of heat-164

Impotence-73, 165, 166, 188, 203, 205, 214, 215, 284, 285

Improves
- blood circulation-34
- sagging skin below eyes-27

Inability to walk-151

Incontinence of Urine-162

Indigestion-5, 9, 73, 133, 134, 136, 149R, 158, 288, 291

Indigestion-gas-163

Infection
- abdomen-184
- ear-8
- eyes-25
- fungal-258
- virus-16

Infectious disease-238

Infertility-11, 248, 279

Inflammation
- colon-295
- legs-6
- mastoid-14

Influenza-193, 211

Injuries
- ankle-284
- brain-15
- head-64
- testicles-289

Insect bite-256

Insomnia-8, 19, 76A, 108B, 113, 114, 194, 242, 246, 272, 274, 275, 284, 285, 290

Intestines
- disorder-14, 146L, 146R, 154, 158, 278
- problem-40, 146R, 243, 277, 278
- large-204
- small-154, 206
- strain-184
- worms-258

Intoxication-39

Iritis-25

Irregularities of
- heart beat-114
- menstruation-164, 165, 166, 209

Irritability-113, 114, 196

Irritation of eyes-16, 26

Itch-276, 277

J

Jaw-272, 274, 275, 284, 285, 290

Jaw lock-35

Jaw tension-35

K

Kidney

Index of Diseses and their Relief Points 141

disease-77, 192, 287
  right-132R
  left-132R
  merdians-153, 284
  stone-270
Knee
  malfunction-260
  pain-52, 246, 248, 278

L

Labour difficulties-258, 285, 293
Laboured breathing-101
Lack of milk-61, 125, 126, 156 (nursing mothers)
Lack of circulation from legs/feet to heart-137
Lack of sex desire-114
Left side body-56L
Legs
  circulation-245
  enlarged-6
  pain-184, 203, 262, 282, 285, 286
  paralysis-246
  pain & sprain-184, 191, 203, 239, 249, 250, 251, 262, 282, 284, 286
  muscles-232, 247
Liver
  problems-125R, 140R, 198, 284
  soothed-17

Long menses period-292
Loss of
  appetite-8, 200
  hearing-8
  consciousness-31, 91, 104
  interest in life-160
  memory-15
  vision-39
  voice-52, 76B
Low blood pressure-3, 10, 274, 275
Low energy-192
Lower backache-151, 183, 184, 192, 202, 205, 206, 236, 238, 267
Lumbar pain-184, 215, 251
Lumbago-238, 251, 252, 262
Lump in throat-160
Lungs
  bloat (Inflammation)-6
  excess fluid-6
  problems-2, 83, 101, 126, 130, 138, 164, 188, 293
Lymph-122L
Lymph abdomen-203

M

Maintenance of life-152
Malfunction of
  heart-260

knee-260
kidney-287

Mastoid inflammation-14

Measles-195, 238, 240

Memory
    deterioration-5, 160
    loss-15

Meningitis-77

Menopause difficulties-151, 203

Menstrual
    cramp-284
    irregularities-164, 165, 166, 209, 254, 276, 277, 278, 280, 284, 290, 292
    pain-65, 274, 275, 276, 277, 284, 290, 296

Mental
    condition-20
    disturbance-158
    fatigue-194
    problems-163
    tension-23, 113, 196

Migraine-4, 7, 10, 11, 12, 13, 19, 33, 61, 75, 76A, 113, 203, 248

Migraine whole body-76A

Motion sickness-8, 108B, 159, 198, 285

Mouth dry-199

Mucous in
bronchi-139L
body-82, 235
colon-139L
heart-139L
intestine-139L, 235
    (from lungs)
nerves-139L

Mumps-35

Muscle cramp-268, 269, 270

Muscle pain-83

N

Nausea-31, 108b, 134, 140, 150, 159, 161, 190, 199, 200, 281, 285, 290, 291

Neck
    pain-7, 65, 167, 187, 255, 257
    stiffness-11, 255
    fatigue-15

Nerves-83, 139R, 208

Nervousness-114, 191

Neuralgia-181, 251, 252

Neurodermatitis-276, 277

Nose/nasal
    blocked/obstruction-1, 13, 16, 23, 24, 26, 30, 76A, 111, 194, 203, 255, 257, 258, 284
    bleeding-1, 2, 4, 11, 12, 13, 29, 30, 31, 76A, 107, 111, 210

Index of Diseses and their Relief Points   143

running-16, 26, 30, 111
Numbness, fingers-90

O

Obesity-113, 243, 247, 276
Old people-83
Old to young-108A
Organs reproductive-35
Over weight-284
Ovaries and tubes-114, 124, 151
Oxygen, absorption-2 (from blood into brain)

P

Pain due to
    Over eating-29, 250, 265
    over drinking-250, 265
Pain in
    abdomen-128, 140, 147, 159, 161, 165, 201L
    ankles-76A, 234, 242, 282, 284
    arms-65, 72, 79, 81
    back-85, 138, 151
    breast-85, 259
    breathing-104, 107, 158, 289
    buttock-236
    chest-74, 83
    cheeks-32
    calf muscle-239, 240
    ear-8
    elbow-63, 76A
    face-27, 32, 35
    fingers-92
    gall bladder-133
    hands-63, 72, 90, 181
    head-81, 201L
    heart-83
    hips-148, 164, 165, 191
    knee-278
    legs-151, 184, 191, 203, 237, 239, 250, 251, 262, 282, 284, 285
    lumbar-184, 215
    lungs-83
    muscles-83
    neck-7, 65, 81, 187
    nerves-83
    prostate-294
    ribs-83, 125, 126, 197, 198, 199
    shoulders-61, 62, 63, 65, 71, 79, 102, 187, 188
    Sides of head-15, 30
    stomach-30, 81, 164, 165
    testicles-290
    toes & feet - 241, 273
    ureter & bladder - 270
    Wrist & hand-89
Painful swelling-238
Palpitation-55, 108B, 112, 114

Pancreas-9, 139R, 143R
Panting-54, 187, 193
Paralysis
    face-27, 30, 31, 34, 76A
    fingers-90
    hand-76A, 103, 112
    legs-201, 240, 246, 248, 278
Pedotic (Potbelly)-116
Perspiration-110, 160
Pharyngitis-104, 107
Pineal problems-6
Pituitary gland-18
Pleural cavity-1
Pneumonia-28
Poisoning tobacco-130
Poor lactation-125
Polyhydrosis-111
Premature ejaculation-73, 76A, 188, 284
Pressure
    high-52, 150, 156, 161, 193, 267
    low-274, 275, 310
Problems of
    abdomen-201L
    ankles-234
    arms-71
    bladder-207
    brain-2, 6, 8, 216
    breathing-22, 65, 101, 104, 289
    bunion-294
    colon-6, 184, 239, 244, 252, 263
    digestion-74, 140, 163, 284
    ears-8
    eyes-61, 266
    feet-137
    gall bladder-199, 203, 248
    heart-5, 125L, 139, 210, 260
    hips-165
    intestines-40, 146R, 277, 243, 278
    kidneys-77, 203
    knee-52, 246, 248
    large intestines-204
    legs-6
    liver-125R, 198
    lungs-2, 101, 293
    lymph-51, 133
    menstrual-165
    mental-163
    nose-1
    pancreas-9, 139R, 143R, 200, 289
    pineal gland-6
    pituitary-6, 18, 210, 281, 293
    sex-285
    small intestines-40, 206, 243
    spinal cord-210
    spleen-200, 289

stomach-2, 5, 210L, 216, 259
thoracic duct-51
thyroid-52, 55, 210
voice-143L

Prostate-105, 164, 167

Psychological disturbance-15

Pulmonary Pain-83

Pus-1

R

Rapid breathing-195

Rashes-76A, 195, 238

Rectal pain-217

Rectum-140

Reproductive hormones-249

Reproductive organs-35, 124, 208, 216, 294

Retention of
  urine-133, 162
  water-154

Rheumatic fever-77

Rheumatoid arthritis-62, 71, 76A, 241, 261

Rib pain-125, 126, 197, 198, 199

Ribs-83, 154, 197

Right side of body-56R

Ringing in ears-15, 33, 34, 203, 215, 254, 268

Running nose-16, 26, 30

S

Scalds-256

Scalp energized-17

Sciatica-110, 184, 236, 237, 238, 239, 240, 242, 250, 251, 284

Serous-133

Serum-133

Sex problems (female)-284, 285

Sexual strength/vigour-183, 192, 203, 205, 275, 280, 285

Shivering-110, 122R, 160, 210

Shock
  electric-29, 31, 64, 109, 114
  others-63, 64, 108B, 113, 122R, 162, 296

Shoulders
  frozen-62
  pain-61, 62, 63, 71, 79, 102, 181, 186, 187, 188
  tension-61

Sickness of
  motion-8, 198
  sea-198

Sinus-1, 16, 23, 24, 27, 30, 31, 76A, 210

Sleeplessness-34, 272

Smooth child delivery-284

Snake bite–112, 251
Sneezing–16, 24, 27, 29, 30, 31
Solar plexus–111, 158, 162
Soothes
    abdomen–17
    gall-bladder–17
    liver–17
Sore
    eyes–16, 76A
    legs–72
    throat–40, 52, 53, 54, 76A, 77, 107
Spasm
    calf–238
    muscles–240
Spasmodic catarrh–16
Spastic condition of
    arms–195
    legs–195
    hips–195
Spermatic cords–151
Spleen–143L, 200, 278, 284, 289
Stiffness
    body–101
    neck–11, 61, 255
Stimulations
    around eyes–24
    food–146R
    intestines–146R
    pituitary–31

Stomach
    ache–24, 26, 134, 144, 145, 164, 182, 191, 197, 259, 261
    cramp–158, 259
    problems–2, 5, 74, 201L, 216
    ulcer–74, 289
Stone kidney–270
Strain/sprain–184, 251
Strained eyes–24, 27
Stroke
    brain–9
    cold–10
    heat–5, 31, 213, 296
    sun–31, 107, 109, 213, 296
Suffocation–105, 110, 160, 269, 286, 296
Sugar control–88, 149R
Sun burn–256
Swallowing
    of air–289
    difficulty–210
Sweating–111, 189
Swelling
    ankles/legs–154, 234, 269
    abdomen–164
    eyes–11, 21, 25
Syncope–31, 295, 296

T

Teeth hurts–11

Temperature-55
Tennis elbow-64, 71, 101
Tension
    abdomen-203
    arm-61
    everyday-194
    eyes-22, 25
    face-26, 27, 30, 32, 36, 76A
    general-36, 191, 194, 249
    hip-203
    lower jaw-35, 38
    mental-10, 23, 87, 196
    neck-22, 286
    shoulders-22, 61, 286
    poor vision-25
    ureter & bladder-270
Testicles
    injury-114, 290
    pain-114, 290
Tetanus-130
Thighs-201L
Throat
    lump-160
    sore-52, 153
Thymus gland-154
Thyroid-52, 55, 106, 210, 247
Tingling head to foot-5
Tinnitus-4, 11, 53, 76A
Tiredness of
    arms-107
    legs-237, 240, 245, 249, 285
    vision-27
Tobacco-130
Tonic for
    elderly people-83, 247
    facial muscles-21, 32
    general health-72, 73, 76A, 83
Toning up of muscles of
    chin-37
    mouth-37
Tonsillitis-35, 76A, 102, 106
Toothache
    lower jaws-35
    upper jaw-33
    both jaw-32, 33, 34, 36, 41, 76A, 80, 87, 91, 113
Toxicity-8
Twisted ankles-234

U

Ulcer
    duodenal-28, 163
    legs-137
    stomach-74, 289
Un-consciousness-104
Ureter-168, 270
Urine retention-133, 162
Urinary problems-165, 203, 248, 284, 286

Uterus-105, 153, 167
Utilization of
    calcium-163
    fat/oil-163
    starch-163
    sugar-163

V

Veins circulation
    to heart-157
    to breast- 122R
    from colon-131R
    from intestines-131R
Velvety swelling-238
Vertigo-103
Virus infection-16
Vision
    blurred-20
    loss-39
    poor-25
    tired-25, 27
Visual disturbances-22, 24, 76A, 203
Vital for body cells-191
Voice
    loss-52, 76B
    problem-143L
Vomiting-11, 108B, 128, 159, 182, 190, 247

W

Warms body-61
Water retention-154, 168
Weak
    body-203
    heart-196
Weight excess-55
Well-being-72, 83
Wet dreams-164, 165, 166, 215
Whiplash-54, 76A, 90, 186
Winter ailments-16
Worms intestine-258
Worries-162
Wound-63, 256, 272, 279
Wrinkles
    chin-38
    eyes-26
    face & neck-19
    lower jaws-35
    mouth-36
    premature-35
    skin-19
Wrist pain-89
Wrist ailment-109

9.
GLOSSARY

A

Abscess – A localized collection of pus in any part of the body, formed by tissue disintegration and surrounded by an inflamed area.

Acne – An inflammatory disease of the oil glands marked by pimples, esp. on the face.

Aerophagia – The abnormal spasmodic swallowing of air - as a symptom of hysteria.

Amino-acids – Organic compounds containing both an amino group (NH_2) and a carboxylic acid group (COOH)– A condition marked by excess amino acids in the blood.

Anemia – A pathological deficiency in the oxygen carrying material of the blood.

Angina – A disease such as croup or diphtheria, in which spasmodic and painful suffocation or spasm occur.

Anus – The excretory opening of the alimentary canal.

Aorta – The main trunk of the systemic arteries carrying blood from the left side of the heart to the arteries of all limbs and organs except the lungs.

Apoplexy – Sudden loss of muscular control, with diminution or loss of sensation and consciousness resulting from rupture or blocking of blood vessels used in the brain.

Appendicitis – Inflammation of the vermiform appendix.

Arthritis – Inflammation of a joint or joints.

Asthma – A chronic reciprocatory disease, often arising from allergies and accompanied by laboured breathing, chest constriction and coughing.

B

Bile – A bitter, alkaline, brownish/greenish yellow liquid secreted by the liver, stored in the gall-bladder and discharged into duodenum, it aids in digestion, chiefly by saponifying fats.

Bile duct – Any of the passages in liver that conveys bile from the liver to the hepatic duct.

Bloat – A swelling.

Bronchus – Either of two main branches of the trachea, leading directly to lungs.

Bruises – To injure without breaking or rupturing.

Bunion – Painful, inflamed swelling of the bursa of big toe.

Bursa – A sac like bodily cavity, esp. one located between joints or at points of friction between moving structures.

Bursitis – Inflammation of a bursa, esp. in the shoulder, elbow or knee joint.

C

Cataract – Opacity of lens or capsule of the eye causing partial or total blindness.

Cervical – Relating to neck or cervix.

Chyle – A thick white or pale-yellow fluid consisting of lymph and finely emulsified fat taken up by the lacteal from the intestine.

Colitis – Inflammation of the mucous membrane of colon.

Colon – Section of large intestines extending from the cecum to the rectum.

Glossary

Common cold – An acute inflammation of the nasal mucous membrane marked by discharge of mucus, sneezing and watering of eyes.

Concussion – A violent jarring, shock. An injury of a soft structure, esp. the brain resulting from a violent blow.

Conjunctivitis – Inflammation of the conjunctiva, the mucous membrane that lines the inner surface of the eyelid and the exposed surface of the eye ball.

Constriction – Becoming narrower or smaller, squeezing.

Contusion – Injury without breaking the skin, bruises.

Cramp – A sudden involuntary muscular contraction causing severe pain, often occurring in leg or shoulder as a result of strain or chill. Partial paralysis of excessively used muscles. Sharp persistent pain in the abdomen.

Croup – A pathological condition affecting the larynx in children marked by respiratory difficulty and a harsh cough.

Crow's feet – Wrinkles formed near the outer corners of the eyes.

Cystitis – Inflammation of the urinary bladder.

D

Depression – The condition of feeling sad or melancholy, inability to concentrate, insomnia, dejection and guilt.

Dermatitis – Skin inflammation.

Diabetes – Any of several metabolic disorders marked by excessive discharge of urine and persistent thirst.

Diarrhoea – Pathologically excessive evacuation of watery faces.

Diphtheria – An acute contagious disease caused by infection by bacillus and marked by the formation of false membrane in the throat and other air passages causing difficulty in breathing, high fever and weakness.

Dizziness – A whirling sensation or feeling a tendency to fall.

Dowager's hump – Back curved by age.

Dropsy – An abnormal accumulation of serous fluid in connective tissues or in serous cavity.

Duodenal – Related to duodenum – the first part of the small intestine.

Dyspnoea – Distressed breathing.

E

Eczema – A non-contagious inflammation of the skin marked mainly by redness, itching and the outbreak of lesions that discharge serous matter and become encrusted and scaly.

Epilepsy – A disorder marked by recurring attacks of motor, sensory or psychic malfunction with or without unconsciousness or convulsive movements.

F

Frigidity – Extremely coldness and persistently averse to sexual relations.

G

Gall-bladder – A small pear-shaped muscular sac located under the right lobe of the liver in which bile secreted by the liver is stored.

Gall-stone – A small, hard, pathological concretion chiefly of cholesterol crystals formed in the gall- bladder or in a bile duct.

Gastritis – Chronic or acute inflammation of the mucous membranl living of the stomach.

Gingivitis – Inflammation of the gums.

Glaucoma – A disease of the eyes marked by high intraocular pressure, damaged optic disc, hardening of the eye ball and partial or complete loss of vision.

Gout – A disturbance of the uric-acid metabolism occurring predominantly in males marked by painful inflammation of the joints, esp. of the feet and hands and arthritic attacks, capable of becoming chronic and producing deformity.

H

Hay – An acute allergic condition of the mucous membrane of the upper respiratory tract and the eyes marked by running nose, sneezing, conjunctivitis and headache often caused by an abnormal sensitivity to certain airborne pollens, esp. of the rag weed and related parts.

Haemophilia – A hereditary plasma coagulation disorder principally affecting males but transmitted by females and marked by excessive, sometimes spontaneous bleeding.

Haemorrhage – Bleeding, esp. copious discharge of blood from the blood vessels.

Haemorrhoid – 1. An itching or painful mass of dilated veins in swollen anal tissue.

2. The pathological condition in which such swollen masses occur.

Hepatic – Of, pertaining or resembling the liver.

Hernia – The protrusion of an organ, organic part of other bodily structure through the wall that normally contains it.

Hic-cough – To have an attack of hiccups.

Hic-cup – A spasm of the diaphragm resulting in a sudden abortive inhalation that is stopped by a spasmodic glottal course.

Hives – Urticaria, a skin condition marked by intensely itching welts and caused by allergic reactions to internal or external agents by foci of infections or by psychic stimulation.

Hoarseness – A husky, grating and low voice.

Hysteria – A neurosis marked by conversion symptoms. – excessive or uncontrollable motion such as fear or panic.

I

Impotence – Incapability of sexual intercourse.

Indigestion – Inability to digest food.

Infection – Invasion by pathogenic micro-organisms of a bodily part in which conditions are favourable for their growth, production of toxins, and subsequent injury to tissues.

Infertility – Incapability of producing child.

Inflammation – Localized heat, redness, swelling, pain, etc. as a result of irritation, injury or infection.

Influenza – An acute infectious viral disease marked by inflammation of reciprocatory tract, fever, muscular pain and irritation in the intestinal tract.

Insomnia – Chronic inability to sleep.

Iritis – Inflammation of the iris of eyes.

Itching – A skin sensation causing a desire to scratch.

K

Kidneys – A pair of structures in the dorsal region of abdominal cavity in vertebrates functioning to maintain proper water balance, regulate acid-base concentration and excrete metabolic waste such as urine.

L

Labour difficulties – Hardships in child birth.

Laboured breathing – Difficult breathing.

Larynx – The upper part of the respiratory tract between pharynx and trachea, having cartilaginous walls containing vocal cords enveloped in folds of the mucous membrane attached to the sides.

Lumbago – A painful, inflammatory rheumatism of the tendons and muscles of lumbar region.

Lumbar – Of or situated in the lower part of the back and sides between the lowest ribs and the pelvis.

Glossary 155

Lymph – A clear transparent, watery or faint yellowish liquid that contains white blood cells and some red blood cells, travels through the lymphatic systems and acts to remove bacteria from tissues to transport fat from intestines and to supply lymphocytes to the blood.

M

Mastoid – The rear portion of the temporal bone on each side of the head behind the ear in man and many other vertebrates.

Measles – An acute, contagious, viral disease usually occurring in childhood and marked by eruption of red spots.

Meningitis – Inflammation of any or all of the meninges of the brain and the spinal cord usually caused by a bacterial infection.

Menopause – The period of cessation of menstruation occurring usually around 45 to 50 years of age.

Migraine – Severe recurrent headache usually affecting only one side of head and marked by sharp pain and often accompanied by nausea.

Motion-sickness – Sickness induced by motion as in travel by air, car, ship or other vehicle and marked by nausea, vomiting and often dizziness.

Mucous – Producing or secreting mucus.

Mucus – The viscous suspension of mucin watery cells and inorganic salts secreted as a protective lubricant coating by glands in the mucous membrane.

Mumps – An acute, inflammatory contagious disease of salivary glands, esp. the parotid and sometimes of the pancreas, ovaries, testes, caused by virus.

N

Nausea – Stomach disturbance marked by a feeling to vomit.

Neuralgia – A sudden outburst of pain along a nerve.

Neuro-dermatitis – Inflammation of skin and nerve.

Numbness – Deprive of the energy to move, paralysis temporarily.

O

Obesity – Extreme fatness due to over eating.

Oedema – An excessive accumulation of serous fluid in the tissues.

Oesophagus – A muscular membranous tube for the passage of food from the pharynx to the stomach.

Osteomyelitis – Inflammation of the bone marrow.

P

Palpitation – Irregular and rapid beating of heart.

Paralysis – Partial or complete inability to move or function a bodily part as a result of injury or disease of its nerve.

Panting – Breathing heavily in short gasps, throbbing, fast pulse.

Perspiration – Abnormal act of perspiring due to some reasons such as despair, excitement, etc.

Pharyngitis – Inflammation of pharynx.

Pharynx – Section of the digestive tract that extends from the nasal cavities to larynx, there becoming continuous with the espohagus.

Pineal – A small elementary glandular body of uncertain function in the brain that is said to be the third eye, an endocrine organ or the seat of the soul.

Pleural cavity – Cavity in the chest enveloping lungs etc.

Pneumonia – Acute chronic disease marked by inflammation of the lungs caused by viruses, bacteria and physical/chemical agents.

Portal-vein – A vein that conducts blood from the digestive organs, spleen, pancreas, and gall-bladder to the liver.

Premature ejaculation – An early and abrupt discharge of seminal fluid.

Glossary

Prostate – A gland in male mammals composed of muscular and glandular tissue that surrounds the urethra at the bladder.

Pulmonary – Of or pertaining to lungs.

Pus – A viscous, yellowish-white fluid formed in infected tissues.

R

Rashes – Skin eruptions or blemish.

Rectal pain – Pain of or near the rectum.

Rectum – Portion of the large intestine between S-shaped bend and canal.

Rheumatic fever – A severe infectious disease occurring chiefly in children marked by fever and painful inflammation of the joints and frequently resulting in permanent damage to the valves of the heart.

Rheumatism – Any of several pathological conditions of the muscles, tendons, joints, bones or nerves marked by discomfort and disability. – Rheumatoid arthritis.

Rheumatoid arthritis – A chronic disease marked by stiffness and inflammation of the joints, weakness, loss of mobility and deformity.

Rheumatoid – Of or resembling rheumatism.

S

Sacrum – A triangular bone made of five fused vertebrae and forming the back-section of the pelvis.

Sarcoma – A malignant tumour arising from non-epithelial connective tissues.

Scalds – Burns with hot liquid/water or steam.

Sciatic nerve – A sensory and motor nerve originating in the sacral plexus and running through the pelvis and upper leg.

Sciatica – Chronic nerve pain in the area of hip or thigh.

Serous – Containing, secreting or resembling serum.

Serum – The clear yellowish fluid obtained by separating blood into its solid and liquid components. Watery fluid such as that found in edema.

Sinus – Disease affecting the sinus membrane.

Sinusitis – Inflammation of sinus membrane.

Sneezing – Expelling air forcibly from the mouth and nose in an explosive spasmodic involuntary action resulting from irritation of the nasal mucosa.

Solar plexus – A large network of sympathetic nerves and ganglia located in the peritoneal cavity behind the stomach and having branching tracts that supply nerves to the abdominal viscera.

Spasm – A sudden involuntary contraction of a muscle or a sudden burst of energy, activity or emotion.

Spasmodic – Pertaining to spasm, convulsive or happening intermittently.

Spastic – Of, pertaining to or marked by spasm.

Spermatic cord – A cord like structure consisting of vas deferens and its accompanying arteries, veins, nerves and lymphatic vessels from the abdominal cavity through the inguinal canal down into the scrotum to the back of the testicle.

Spermatic – Of, pertaining to or resembling sperm.

Spleen – One of the largest lymphoid structures in human beings, a visceral organ composed of a white pulp of lymphatic nodules and tissues and a red pulp of vinous sinusoid in a framework of fibrous partitions lying on the left side below the diaphragm, functioning as a blood filter and blood storage.

Sprain – A painful wrenching or laceration of the ligament of a joint.

Sternum – A long flat bone artificially with the cartilages and forming the support of most of the ribs, collar bone, etc.

Glossary

Syncope – A brief loss of consciousness caused by transient anemia.

T

Tennis elbow– Strain and pain in the elbow due to swing which has not worked in tennis.

Tetanus – An acute often fatal infections disease caused by a bacillus that generally enter the body through wounds marked by rigidity and spasmodic contraction of the voluntary muscles.

Thoracic duct – The main duct of the lymphatic system ascending along the spinal cord and discharging into the venous system.

Thymus – A ductless gland like structure situated just behind the top of sternum, that plays some part in building resistance to disease but is usually vestigial in adults after reaching its maximum development during early childhood.

Thyroid gland – A two lobed endocrine gland found in all vertebrates located in front of and on either side of the trachea in humans and producing the hormone thyroxin.

Tonsillitis – Inflammation of the tonsils.

Toxicity – A poisonous substance.

U

Ulcer – An inflammatory, often supur-ating lesion on the skin or an internal mucous surface of the body resulting in necrosis of the tissue.

Ureter – The long narrow duct that conveys urine from the kidney to the urinary bladder.

V

Vein – A vessel transporting blood towards heart.

Velvety swelling – Swelling as soft & smooth as velvet.

Venous – Of or pertaining to veins.

Vermiform – Resembling or having the shape of a worm.

W

Whiplash – An injury to cervical spine caused by an abrupt jerking motion of the head either backward or forward.

Writer's cramp – A cramp chiefly affecting the muscles of the thumb and two adjacent fingers of the thumb due to prolonged writing.

BIBLIOGRAPHY

A Complete book of Acupuncture	by Dr. Stephen Thomas Chang. 1976 – Celestial Arts, Berkeley, CA.
A Layman's Guide to Acupuncture	By Yoshio Manaka, M.D. & Ian A. Urquhart, Ph. D., 1972 – Weatherhill, N.Y., Tokyo.
Aapka Arogya Aapke Hath Main	Acupressure Padyati (Reflexology) by Divendra Vora, 1982 Rev. Ed. 1990
Acupressure (Anybody Can Do It)	By Leon A. Hart, 1977 – Lynn Mark Library, N.Y.
Acupressure, Face Lift	by Lindsay Wagner, 1986
Back Pains, Quick Relief without Drugs	by Dr. Howard D. Kurland, M.D., 1981.
Breathing Easy	by Gnell Subak – Sharpe, James V. Warren, M.D., 1988 – Doubleday, N.Y.
Chinese Massage	by Hortley and Mark, 1987
Essentials of Human Anatomy and Physiology	by Elaine Nicpon Marieb, 1984
Finger Acupressure	by Pedro chan, 1989
Freedom From Pain Through Acupressure	by Frank Z. Warren, 1976

Heeling Massage technique	by frances M. Tappan
Helping Yourself With Natural Remedies	by Terry Willard, Ph.D., 1951
High Energy	by Rob Krakovitz, M.D., 1986 – J.P. Tracher, Inc., L.A.
Home Nursing	by Diana Hastings, RGN, RCNT, 1987 – Barron's Educational Series, Inc. N.Y.
Homeopathic Medicine At Home	by Maesimund B. Panos, M.D. and Jane Heimlich, 1987 – J.P. Tracher, Inc., L.A.
Homeopathy	by Sarah Richardson, 1989
Massage at Your Finger Tips	by Science Life Books, 1984 Revised by E.R. Triance
Modern Chinese Acupuncture	by G.T. Lewith, M.A., M.R.C.G.P., M.R.C.P. and N.R. Lewith MCSP, 1983 – Thorsons Publishers, Inc., N.Y.
No Drug Guide to Better Health	by Eleonore Blaurock Bush., Ph.D., 1984 with Berud W. Bush, D.C.
Pediatrics for parents (A Guide to Child Health)	By H. Winter Griffith, M.D., Howard Mofenson, M.D. - Mosby Co., St. Louis (Copy Right) Thomas A. Manning, N.Y. - Joseph Greensher, M.D., Arnold Greensher, M.D.
Quick Headache Relief Without Drugs	by Dr. Howard D. Kurland, M.D., 1977
Reflexology	by Nieola M. Hall, 1986
Relax with Self Therapy/Ease	by Bonnie Pendleton and Betty Mehling, 1984

Self-Help-OSTEOPATHY	by Robert Bowden, 1988
Seven Keys of Color Healing	by Roland Hunt, 1982
Shiatzu	by Yukiko Irwin with James Wagenvoord, 1976 – J. B. Lippincott Co., Philadelphia & N.Y.
Shiatzu – Japanese Finger Pressure Therapy	by William Schultz – Bell Publishing Co., N.Y.
The Human Body	by Ruth Dowling Brush, M.D. and Bertel Brumn, M.D. – Random House, N.Y.
The Reflexology Work-Out	by Stephanie Rick, 1986
Therepeutic Touch	by Dolores Krieger, Ph.D., RN, 1987
Up From Depression	by Leonard Cammer, M.D., 1969 – Simon and Schuster, N.Y.
Vitamin Book	by Harold M Silverman, Pharm D., 1985 – Bartan Books Inc., 666 5th Ave., N.Y.-10103
Wake up ! You're Alive	by Arnold Fox, M.D. and Barry Fox, 1988 – Health Communications, Inc., Fl.
Your Thyroid	by Lawrance C Wood, M.D., FACP, 1982 – Ballantine Books, Random House Inc., N.Y.

A wide variety of Books on the following subjects by Indian and Foreign Authors are also available with us:

- Acupressure and Reflexology
- Acupuncture
- Aroma Therapy
- Astrology and Palmistry
- Ayurveda and Herbal Medicine
- Bach Flower Remedies
- Biochemistry
- Crystal and Gem Therapy
- Dowsing - Pendulum
- Feng Shui
- Health Care
- Holistic Medicine
- Homoeopathy
- Hypnosis
- Iridology
- Juice and Food Therapy
- Magnetotherapy
- Medical Dictionary
- Nature Cure
- Pet Animals
- Pranic Healing
- Reiki and Spiritualism
- Tai Chi
- Tarot
- Urine Therapy
- Vaastu
- Yoga

A detailed catalogue of books is available with B. Jain Publishers (P) Ltd.

Ph: 2358 0800, 2358 1100, 2358 1300, 2358 3100
Fax: 011-2358 0471; Email: bjain@vsnl.com
Website: www.bjainbooks.com

on request.

Acupressure, Magnetic and Feng Shui gadgets are also available.